A Man's Guide to a
Nursing Career

Chad E. O'Lynn, PhD, RN, RA is an assistant professor of nursing at the University of Portland. He has been a clinical nurse specialist and adult nurse practitioner, serving neuroscience and geriatric populations. He has been a full-time educator and consultant since 2002. Dr. O'Lynn's research has examined rural health, men's health, and the dedicated education unit model for clinical education. However, he is most known for his research on men in nursing, particularly male nursing students. He was the lead editor for *Men in Nursing: History, Challenges, and Opportunities* (2007, Springer Publishing), the first academic book devoted solely to men in nursing. He is a national speaker on men in nursing and has held leadership positions in the American Assembly for Men in Nursing. He is also a registered aromatherapist. Dr. Lynn obtained his PhD from the Oregon Health & Sciences University, Portland, in 2006.

A Man's Guide to a Nursing Career

Chad E. O'Lynn, PhD, RN, RA

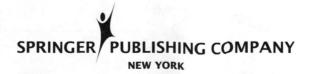

SPRINGER PUBLISHING COMPANY
NEW YORK

Copyright © 2013 Springer Publishing Company, LLC

Springer Publishing Company, LLC
11 West 42nd Street
New York, NY 10036
www.springerpub.com

Acquisitions Editor: Allan Graubard
Production Editor: Joseph Stubenrauch
Composition: Exeter Premedia Services Private Ltd.

ISBN: 978-0-8261-0685-8
E-book ISBN: 978-0-8261-0686-5
13 14 15/ 5 4 3 2

The author and the publisher of this Work have made every effort to use sources believed to be reliable to provide information that is accurate and compatible with the standards generally accepted at the time of publication. The author and publisher shall not be liable for any special, consequential, or exemplary damages resulting, in whole or in part, from the readers' use of, or reliance on, the information contained in this book. The publisher has no responsibility for the persistence or accuracy of URLs for external or third-party Internet websites referred to in this publication and does not guarantee that any content on such websites is, or will remain, accurate or appropriate.

Library of Congress Cataloging-in-Publication Data
A man's guide to a nursing career / Chad E. O'Lynn.
     p. ; cm.
   Includes bibliographical references.
   ISBN 978-0-8261-0685-8—ISBN 978-0-8261-0686-5 (e-book)
   I. Title.
   [DNLM: 1. Nurses, Male.   2. Career Choice.   3. Nursing.   4. Vocational Guidance. WY 191]
   610.73023—dc23

                                                              2012030583

Printed in the United States of America by Bang Printing.

With great deference,
I dedicate this book to Dr. Russell "Gene" Tranbarger.
Dr. Tranbarger has devoted his 50-plus or -minus-year career
to supporting the recruitment
and professional development of men in nursing.
His wisdom, gentle motivation, willingness to give,
compassion, and his laughter make him
an incomparable educator, administrator, and role model.
I am forever grateful for his mentorship
and partnership on our book,
Men in Nursing: History, Challenges,
and Opportunities *(2007, Springer Publishing).*
Without a doubt, I will realize success
if I attain just a fraction of his accomplishments.

Contents

Contributors

Stacey Boatright, MA has dedicated her entire professional career to helping nursing students achieve their educational and professional goals. She has been a staff member at the University of Portland School of Nursing since 2001 and has been the graduate program counselor and grant manager since 2005. In her role, she is responsible for recruiting, admission, orientation, academic advising, and general student assistance for all graduate nursing programs and students. In addition, Boatright manages federal and private grants that support programs and students in the School of Nursing. She received an MA from the University of Portland in 2009.

Renee G. Heath, PhD has studied power and decision-making in organizations' collaborating stakeholder groups since 1997. She teaches graduate- and undergraduate-level communication courses for the University of Portland in Communication Studies and the MBA program. Her work on collaboration and dialogue has been published in major communication journals including the *Journal of Applied Communication Research, Management Communication Quarterly,* and the *Journal of Business Communication.* Dr. Heath worked as the development director of the Providence Benedictine Nursing Center and has maintained a group fitness certification from the American Council of Exercise since 1996. She consults and trains diverse groups including professionals in the Pamplin Business School (University of Portland) Executive Education program. Dr. Heath was awarded a PhD by the University of Colorado, Boulder, in 2005.

Foreword

In 1998, I volunteered to help with a classroom party in my daughter Katharine's kindergarten class. Her teacher introduced me to the class as Mr. Lecher. She said that I was a nurse who worked at Cincinnati Children's Hospital Medical Center. Both the boys and girls started saying things like, "You can't be a nurse because you're not Katharine's mom." Four years later, I volunteered in my son Nick's first grade class. This time, the teacher introduced me by saying, "Class, this is Nick's dad, Mr. Lecher. He is a nurse at Children's Hospital." Again the first grade boys and girls began saying that dads can't be nurses. Then in 2011, my 17-year-old daughter was volunteering as a teacher's assistant with a summer religious education program at our church with children soon-to-be third-graders. I stopped by for a visit one day wearing my hospital identification badge. I also had a second badge with "RN" printed on it in large letters. I was not there very long when one of the boys saw my badge and said, "You can't be a nurse, only ladies can be nurses."

These three personal anecdotes highlight why *A Man's Guide to a Nursing Career* is needed. Currently, American children learn messages at a very early age that suggest that men cannot be nurses. These messages must change. Men have much to offer as nurses. In 2010, the Institute of Medicine proclaimed that the nursing workforce must become more diverse in terms of gender, race, and ethnicity if health care quality is to be realized. And although more men are entering nursing, the pace of increase has been glacially slow. This book will be an important tool in recruiting and retaining more men in nursing.

This book serves as a guide for young men, their families, and friends. Parents, other family members, and friends are key sources of support who also have questions. Not that long ago a father and son were referred to me to talk about nursing. The student was on the verge of declining a full scholarship to play football at a regional university. He said that his heart was no longer in football and that he wanted to become a nurse instead like his aunt. He wanted to work with and help people. The father's first question to me was "Will my son be okay if he goes to school and becomes a nurse?" I reassured them both that a nursing education and license will provide career opportunities and benefits for a lifetime. Fortunately, the student is now working at Cincinnati Children's Hospital and is about half way through his program to earn his Bachelor of Science in Nursing (BSN) degree. This book could be a wonderful resource for families like his as they ask the question, "Will it be okay?"

I want to congratulate Chad O'Lynn for putting together this book about men in nursing. The first section provides a comprehensive background on the opportunities for men in nursing, male role models, and continued gender challenges. The next section describes how to be successful at getting in and staying in nursing school and discusses the gender differences related to caring and compassion. Finally, the last section gives the reader successful strategies to get an RN license, the first job, working in a gender-imbalanced culture, and career progression and advancement. If you are a young man with this book in hand, read it and pursue your first nursing degree. If you are a parent with gender-related questions about your son becoming a nurse, don't worry. We need more men in nursing, and the career opportunities are endless. And if you are a new nurse, pay attention to the advice given on how to strengthen your new career.

As a parent and a man in nursing, it is my hope that in the future, it will be natural for boys to tell their parents, teachers, and friends that they want to be a nurse when they grow up. This book, along with organizations such as the American Assembly for Men in Nursing (www.aamn.org) and supportive employers like Cincinnati Children's Hospital Medical Center, will help nursing's journey to become more diverse, inclusive, and one day gender-balanced. With more men in nursing, when dad the nurse comes to visit the first grade class, funny looks will be nothing more than a distant memory.

William T. Lecher, RN, MS, MBA, NE-BC
President, American Assembly for Men in Nursing
Senior Clinical Director, Cincinnati Children's Hospital Medical Center

Preface

In 2001, I attended my first conference of the American Assembly for Men in Nursing (AAMN) in Austin, Texas. The gathering was small; many people were unable to come due to the travel problems following the 9/11 terrorist attacks that had occurred just a few weeks prior to the conference. A few scheduled presenters were unable to attend, so there were long breaks between conference sessions. These breaks were filled with networking and extended discussions of issues. Most of the issues related to the challenges of being a man in nursing. I was amazed by some of the stories of hardship and perseverance these men shared. Although I had been a nurse for 15 years at that point, I thought gender issues in nursing only applied to me and just a few other men. I had no idea that every man probably had a story to tell. Then again, I had never before been in a room with so many other male nurses.

During the conference, one nurse recently out of school commented that information sessions were valuable and would have been helpful as he struggled through some issues while a student. He asked if there was a book about men in nursing. No one in the room knew of any, to which he replied, "Well, someone ought to write a book." I found this challenge provocative, and two years later, asked a colleague and mentor, Dr. Russell Tranbarger, to partner with me in editing the first academic textbook on men in nursing (*Men in Nursing: History, Challenges, and Opportunities*, Springer Publishing, 2007).

The book received much praise as it clearly addressed a gap in the literature. However, the book also received some criticism, mostly due to its academic and theoretical tone. In 2009, while attending a men in nursing conference at Monterey Peninsula College in California, a few nursing students approached me after a presentation I had given. They told me that they had read parts of the book and found it valuable, but preferred the practical information they were getting at the conference. They told me that they needed information that they could easily apply to their situations right now. One student said, "Some guys I know couldn't come today. It would be great if this stuff was written down." I left thinking that a new type of book was needed for young men in nursing. Coincidentally, shortly afterward, I was approached by Springer about preparing a second edition to our book. I told the representative that there was not enough new information and research to warrant a second edition, but I did share with him the comments I had received from the students in Monterey. The plan for this second book was then born. I took some initial ideas and ran them by my students and male colleagues. Their input on what type of book should be written was instrumental in creating the book you now have in your hands.

The audience for this book is twofold. Young men, ages 16 to 25, who are considering a career in nursing or are currently matriculated as nursing students, will find this book helpful and illuminating; their families and friends included. Nurses currently in practice will also gain from the book as it discusses issues specific to male nurses and nursing in a predominantly female profession. In this light, I have kept technical terms and jargon to a minimum. The information presented is well-researched yet concise. Throughout are personal anecdotes and instructions, when appropriate, so that the book is grounded and clear. The content also is laid out to match the path of a new career in nursing, from thinking about becoming a nurse up to the first couple of years in nursing practice. I have divided the book into three sections that roughly correspond to the three major sections of this early career path.

The first section covers that period of time when you are considering a career in nursing, which I call *Why Men? Why Nursing? Why Now?* Chapter 1 gives an overview of the benefits and opportunities awaiting you in nursing. Some of these benefits are tangible, such as good pay and job security. Others are less tangible, but nonetheless, just as important, such as respect and job satisfaction. I present a case to strive for your bachelor's degree in this chapter and introduce the common advanced roles that can take your career into stimulating and fulfilling directions. Chapter 2 gives an overview of the history of men in nursing. This topic was covered more fully in the previous book, but that chapter lacked clear identification of historical role models. A lack of role models contributes to a sense of isolation. Here, I cover men's history through brief stories of historical and modern role models. Since some may consider historical role models irrelevant to today's modern world, I follow each story with the lessons today's men can learn from these early nursing leaders. This format, history via male role models and the lessons they teach us, makes this chapter quite unique. In Chapter 3, I provide a brief explanation why some have had, and may still have, discomfort with the presence of men in nursing. When many of us became nurses, we naively expected other nurses to recognize our energy and talent, and welcome us into the profession with open arms. This welcome often happened. Sometimes it did not simply because we were men. This negative response may serve as a source of friction and self-doubt—something that is rarely discussed in nursing school. Chapter 3 attempts to provide you with some background and understanding so that you may respond positively to any unwelcome reception.

The next section is titled *Making it Happen*, and covers the preparation and educational period of becoming a nurse. In Chapter 4, my insightful and experienced colleague, Stacey Boatright, discusses the best strategies of how to get into nursing school. To the surprise of many students, becoming a nurse isn't as easy as just signing up for nursing classes at the local

college or university. In reality, there are a limited number of slots in nursing school, so admission is quite competitive. You will find Stacey's advice
invaluable. Chapter 5 covers the barriers you might encounter once you are
a nursing student. Every student has some challenges, but nursing students
have a very different experience than most college students. The demands
and rigor of a nursing education makes the life of a nursing student stressful. Some challenges can be so intense that they become a potential barrier
to finishing school and becoming a nurse. Examination of these barriers has
been an important component of my own research. In Chapter 5, I discuss
potential barriers that any nursing student might face, but then direct your
attention to barriers that are unique to male nursing students. I also provide
tips on how to minimize these barriers so that your nursing student journey
can be as productive as possible. In Chapter 6, I discuss the all-important
topic of caring and touch. No other issues are as uncomfortable for men as
these two, yet they are rarely covered in much depth in nursing school. How
nurses have displayed caring and have used touch historically has fed into a
feminine stereotype of nursing that challenges men. In this chapter, I argue
that there are many different and equal ways to demonstrate care, not just
the touchy-feely style we associate with women. I also provide tips on how
to touch patients' bodies comfortably and in a manner that communicates
respect and professionalism.

The last section is titled *The Eagle Has Landed! Working as a Registered
Nurse* and covers the transition period between nursing school and the first
two years of professional practice. This time period is extremely stressful.
Often, there is a disconnect between what the former nursing student has
envisioned for himself as a nurse and the reality of working as a nurse in a
setting where he must now shoulder responsibilities independently. Again, I
believe men have a unique journey during this transition, particularly as they
try to socialize into the culture of nursing. In Chapter 7, I explain how to get
your nursing license, which first requires that you pass the licensure exam
(NCLEX-RN®). I provide tips on how to pass this exam on the first attempt,
followed by tips on getting that first nursing job. The latter is especially
important today, since nursing jobs are not as plentiful for many new graduates as they were in different economic times. For Chapter 8, I invited my
colleague Renee Heath to share her expertise on communication. Some may
think that communication is not so important to warrant a full chapter on the
topic, but I strongly disagree. The reality is that nursing is overwhelmingly
female, and male–female challenges with communication are well-known.
Also, there is an increased emphasis on the importance of teamwork in
health care settings. Teamwork requires excellent communication. Many men
have told me that their biggest on-the-job challenge is communicating and
working with some of their female coworkers. In this chapter, Renee doesn't
dwell excessively on male-versus-female differences. Instead, Renee focuses
on how to best work with team members who have different assumptions
about communication. Lastly, Chapter 9 sends you off into your career with
a discussion of professional development. The need to continue to learn and
grow continues throughout your career. Development plans must be started
early in your career if you are going to avoid stagnation and burnout. In this

chapter, I discuss how to obtain and work with mentors. I also instruct you to return the favor by becoming a mentor to the nurses that follow you. I also touch on leadership development. To become an effective leader in today's nursing world, you must adopt new perspectives that include an understanding of systems and chaos. You may have heard about these perspectives in your nursing courses, but systems issues and chaos can hit you hard once you begin working as a nurse. I encourage you to start to understand these perspectives so that you can affect change and improvement in your own practice and in the settings in which you work.

And one last note: in a few appropriate places in this book, I have very intentionally used the pronoun *he* to refer to a generic nurse. A common irritation for men in nursing is the use of *she* when referring to the generic nurse. Following the practice of my feminist friends who intentionally use *she* in male-dominated contexts in order to raise the reader's awareness of gender discrimination, the use of *he* in this book seems appropriate. My intent by doing this is not to exclude or offend my female readers.

Putting this book together has been like a long-term relationship. At times I have embraced the content with passion. At other times, I have had to take some cooling-off periods and put the book aside for a few months. But I have never lost sight of the conversations I have had with men in nursing. So here is this book. It's designed to be rather brief, accessible, and provide easy-to-apply information to your personal situation. The focus of this book is on the early portions of your nursing career, a time filled with risk and doubt. Although you will find many other books to guide your career journey once you have become a nurse, I trust that you will keep this book as a reference, especially as you advise and mentor young men as they start their own journeys as nurses.

Fear not to spread your wings. Use them to soar to new heights and to protect those entrusted in your care. Happy reading!

Acknowledgments

I am deeply grateful to my colleagues Renee Heath and Stacey Boatright, who generously contributed their expertise to this book. I am inspired by the numerous men in nursing school who persevere despite adversity in their journeys. I thank Allan Graubard, Executive Editor, Springer Publishing, for giving me such a generous timeline to complete my work. And most importantly, I owe much to my partner Doug, for his love and understanding of my many late nights at the computer. You really are the best!

ONE

What Can Nursing Bring to You?

I probably don't have to tell you that nursing is an excellent career choice. Even during the recent recession, employment in health care remained strong. In fact, it has been one of the few industries that has continued to hire new employees, making it rather recession-proof. Of all health care careers, nursing offers the most flexibility and opportunities. In 2008, there were over 3 million nurses in the United States (U.S. Department of Health and Human Services [USDHS], 2010), making them the largest group of professionals in health care (Dohm & Shniper, 2007). And even though more people are becoming nurses, there continues to be a shortage of nurses that will worsen, especially as older nurses retire (American Association of Colleges of Nursing [AACN], 2011a; Auerbach, Buerhaus, & Staiger, 2011; Buerhaus & Auerbach, 2011). In fact, the job growth for registered nurses from 2010 to 2020 is believed to be 26%, higher than the average for all occupations (Bureau of Labor Statistics, U.S. Department of Labor [BLS], 2012a). The ongoing demand for nurses has captured the attention of the media. News reports, public service announcements, and ad campaigns have become common, all in an effort grow the nursing workforce. Perhaps you have seen some of these. They mention the good pay, professional opportunities, and job satisfaction. But there are other benefits of becoming a nurse. And nursing for men has never been better.

JOB SECURITY

The nursing shortage practically guarantees job security, something important to consider in these tough economic times. Even though it is harder for some nurses to find their ideal job right after school (see Chapter 7), the vast majority of graduating nursing students find jobs in just a short period of time. As the economy recovers from the recent recession, nurses will be in higher demand. If current projections hold true, there will be a need for an additional 712,000 nurses by 2020, and possibly as many as 3 million more nurses by 2030 (Auerbach et al., 2011; BLS, 2012a). These numbers don't include the nurses that will be needed to replace nurses who will retire in the upcoming years. It is unlikely that this need will be met if current levels of nursing students remain stable. All the experts agree; the employment picture for nurses looks bright.

ATTRACTIVE SALARIES

With a shortage of nurses, working nurses command better salaries than many other occupations. Also, nursing salaries continued to rise even during the recession. The average salary for a registered nurse in May 2011 was $69,110 per year, or $33.23 per hour (BLS, 2012b). Compare this salary with the average salaries of high-school teachers ($56,260), police officers ($56,260), retail store managers ($40,630), and general construction laborers ($34,170). Keep in mind that salaries vary depending upon the employer, experience, and education of the nurse, and the nursing specialty. Nurses often earn extra money for working nights, weekends, holidays, and overtime. Salaries vary in different locations. For example, nurses earn the highest average salary in California ($90,860) but the lowest in Iowa ($53,300), though new nurses should expect to earn less than advanced practice nurses with many years of experience. Still, nurses typically earn an attractive salary that can support their families.

JOB SATISFACTION

Attractive salaries contribute to high levels of satisfaction among nurses, but other factors count too. For example, relationships with coworkers and management, ability to make independent decisions, opportunities for advancement, workload, hours, health benefits, and many other components of the job contribute to a nurse's level of job satisfaction. Sometimes, these factors are more important than money. For example, nurses who work the night shift can make more money than their day shift colleagues, but night shift work often interferes with family responsibilities and social schedules. In Oregon, nurses who worked in hospitals were more satisfied with their salaries and relationships with their bosses than were nurses who worked in other settings, but nonhospital nurses were more satisfied with the safety of their workplaces, quality of care they could provide patients, personal independence, and their relationships with their patients (Oregon Center for Nursing, 2010). Overall, nonhospital nurses were more satisfied with their jobs than were hospital nurses. These findings were a little different nationally. In total, 79.8% of hospital nurses were satisfied with their jobs and 73.8% of nonhospital nurses were satisfied with their jobs (USDHHS, 2010). Still, these are very high rates of satisfaction. Both in Oregon and nationally, nursing job satisfaction has increased in recent years.

RESPECT

I probably don't need to convince you that the nursing profession is honorable and worthy of respect. Otherwise, you wouldn't be reading this book. But your high regard of nursing is shared by others. Each year since 1977, the Gallup Corporation surveyed the general public about how they rate various professions on honesty and ethical standards. In 1999, they added nurses to the list of professions. The public has rated nursing as the top profession every year since except for 2001, when the Gallup surveyors added firefighters to list following the 9/11 tragedy. Nurses have always been rated higher than doctors, pharmacists, teachers, judges, and the clergy in terms of honesty and ethical behavior. Better yet, the public's high ratings have remained consistent over the years (Gallup, 2012). There are several implications for these high ratings. First, becoming a nurse commands respect. You may get a little ribbing from friends or family who think nursing is women's work (see Chapters 2, 3, 5, and 6), but no one can deny that your career choice is a worthy one. Second, as a nurse, your patients will rely on you for information, for service, and for action. You have their trust, for the most part, simply by having the initials "RN" (registered nurse) after your name. Third, since patients have so many needs, you will find many rewards and much satisfaction knowing that your actions are appreciated by so many. And fourth, the public trusts nurses to lead the way for better health care reform by ensuring that caring, comfort, and patient needs are not forgotten in any changes to the system (IOM, 2011).

OPPORTUNITIES

With such demand, attractive wages, job satisfaction, and public respect, it's no wonder why nursing is so attractive. In addition to these benefits, there are numerous opportunities for nurses to advance and/or refresh their careers. Nursing overflows with different roles, specialties, and work settings, so much so that I tell students there is no reason why a nurse should feel like he is in a rut. With additional training or with a return to school, nurses can change their careers to better match their needs. Few professions offer such variety.

Certified Nursing Assistant, Licensed Practical Nurse / Licensed Vocational Nurse

Most nursing opportunities are available for RNs. There are, however, two other nursing roles that I must mention. First is the certified nursing assistant (CNA). CNAs work under the supervision of other nurses. They provide many direct nursing services to patients in hospitals, clinics, care facilities, and sometimes in patients' homes. CNAs primarily provide assistance with personal tasks (such as hygiene, dressing, and exercise) and health monitoring (such as measuring blood pressure). The range of services CNAs may provide differs from state to state and among employers, but CNAs sometimes give medications and treatments (such as wound care). Our health care system relies heavily on CNAs for this important work. Many CNAs find their work rewarding since they can often develop strong connections with their patients. Many nursing students work as CNAs to further develop their nursing skills. Others work as CNAs as an introduction to nursing. CNAs usually must complete a training course that lasts from several weeks to a few months. These courses are provided by employers, community colleges, or private technical schools. If you have questions whether nursing is the right career for you, I strongly recommend working as a CNA to experience nursing from the inside.

Another role in nursing is the licensed practical nurse or licensed vocational nurse (LPN/LVN). These nurses provide a wider range of services than do CNAs and work generally with much more independence. Typically, LPN/LVNs work under the supervision of the RN or the doctor. LPN/LVNs work in all health care settings and may take supervisory roles in some settings. Depending upon the state, many LPN/LVNs can provide most of the same services as an RN; however, only the RN has full authority (and responsibility) for developing plans of care that are provided to patients. LPN/LVNs carry out plans of care, and assist in revising or updating these plans based on their keen observation skills and meticulous record-keeping (LPNtranining. org, 2012). LPN/LVNs must take courses from local community colleges or technical schools, though most are not required to earn a college degree in order to get their LPN/LVN license.

Pathways to the RN License

Most opportunities in nursing require that you first become an RN. All states require that you complete an approved educational program and pass a licensure exam to become an RN (see Chapter 7). Most nurses earn a college degree. There are four types of educational programs that allow you to get your RN license: diploma, associate's degree (ADN), bachelor's degree (BSN), and the more recent alternative graduate pathways (Raines & Taglaireni, 2008). Diploma programs traditionally were offered by hospitals, but now most are offered jointly by a health care institution and a college. Typically, graduates of these programs do not earn a college degree. The number of these programs has dropped greatly since 1965, when the American Nurses Association recommended that diploma programs move to the college and university system. ADN programs are offered by community and private colleges. Their emphasis in the past had been on teaching students the technical skills of direct nursing care, but many now provide coursework covering leadership, policy, quality improvement, and other professional topics. Interestingly, some refer to these programs as "two-year programs," even though most students require up to three or more years to complete all the required coursework. The BSN program is offered at four-year colleges and universities, and prepares students to work in all health care settings in the widest variety of RN roles. Students learn all the content offered by ADN programs, plus additional education in the humanities, management, and professional practice. And finally, the alternate graduate pathway program was developed to offer students who have a nonnursing bachelor's degree an option to become nurses without starting school over again. Graduates of these programs earn a bachelor's degree in nursing and become nurses and/or earn a graduate nursing degree as well. These programs vary from school to school, but they often offer the undergraduate nursing content at an accelerated pace. These programs prepare students for a variety of roles, including advanced nursing roles.

The multiple paths of becoming an RN have been a source of controversy for many decades. The reasons for the different paths are complex and intertwined with the history of modern nursing. Generally speaking, different paths emerged as educational philosophies changed, as nursing became a more developed profession, as health care became more advanced and complex, and as a means to sustain an adequate number of nurses in times of labor shortages. Today, the primary *benefit* of the different paths is flexibility in options of becoming an RN. Based on your personal finances, schedules, and time constraints, you may choose one path over another. Conversely, the primary *problem* created by different paths is the lack of consistency over the educational preparation of nurses. For many years, there have been intense debates within nursing to establish a minimum RN education requirement. Unlike other health care professions, nursing has been unable to resolve the differences within its ranks. (My belief is that nursing was unable to make bold decisions in fear of upsetting colleagues and employers.) The intensity of the debate lessened in the latter part of the 20th century, as nurses adopted an agree-to-disagree attitude. This attitude, however, hasn't solved the core problem.

In recent years, most health professions recognized that the bachelor's degree was the *minimum* educational requirement for professional practice, with many even requiring graduate degrees. In many clinical settings, nurses have the lowest level of education compared to other health professions. This can make it more difficult for nurses to be treated as equal members of the health care team. More important, less education may also hamper patient care. In several well-publicized studies, RNs with lower levels of education were associated with more negative outcomes for patients, including death, in hospital settings (Aiken, Clarke, Cheung, Sloane, & Siber, 2003; Friese, Lake, Aiken, Silber, & Sochalski, 2008; Kendall-Gallagher, Aiken, Sloane, & Cimiotti, 2011). The findings from Aiken et al.'s 2003 study were confirmed five years later. The researchers found that for every 10% increase in BSN-prepared nurses on staff, hospital risk of death dropped by 4% (Aiken Clarke, Sloane, Lake, & Cheney, 2008).

These studies have been criticized. Good nursing care is provided by all types of nurses in all types of clinical settings. Still, there is a common sense perspective that more education will benefit nurses and their patients. Perhaps the extensive work by the Institute of Medicine (IOM) has convinced nursing to move toward the bachelor's degree as the minimum requirement for RNs better than has these studies. The highly respected IOM has published ground-breaking reports for over 20 years, which have significantly influenced reforms to improve the safety and quality of health care. Their reports described the new responsibilities of nurses and the increased education they will need to meet the challenges of tomorrow. The IOM recommended that at least 80% of all nurses have their BSN degrees by 2020

(IOM, 2011). Their recommendations carry much clout, so much so that the Tri-Council for Nursing (a network of nursing leadership, policy, and education organizations) stated

> Current healthcare reform initiatives call for a nursing workforce that integrates evidence-based clinical knowledge and research with effective communication and leadership skills. These competencies require increased education at all levels....Without a more educated nursing workforce, the nation's health will be further at risk. (AACN, 2010, para. 2)

Although the Council stopped short of recommending a *requirement* of a bachelor's degree, it did acknowledge the need to increase the number of BSN nurses and called for the development of education programs and policies to make it easier for nurses to earn their bachelor's degrees.

Some employers are taking a bolder stance. The U.S. military now requires all active duty nurses in the nurse corps to have a bachelor's degree. The U.S. Public Health Service requires commissioned officers to have a bachelor's degree. The Veteran's Administration will no longer grant promotions beyond entry level to nurses who do not have a bachelor's degree. The nation's magnet hospitals (hospitals recognized for superior nursing quality and patient care) will require that all nurse managers have a bachelor's or graduate degree by 2013 and have plans in place to achieve 80% of their nurses to have bachelor's degrees by 2020. Since many of these hospitals have rates currently lower than 80%, some have stopped hiring nurses who do not have a bachelor's degree (Anna Maria College, 2012).

Even further, New York and New Jersey have introduced proposals to require all new nurses get their BSN degrees within 10 years of graduation if they do not already have one (AACN, 2012a). Other states are considering similar proposals. Such requirements are increasing the number of students enrolled in BSN programs and in ADN-to-BSN completion programs. AACN (2011a) reported that BSN enrollment has increased every year since 2002, and that enrollment in completion programs jumped 13.4% between 2010 and 2011. Still, aggressive action will be needed if the IOM goal of a BSN-prepared workforce is to be realized. Employers, nursing leaders, nursing organizations, and schools of nursing will need to work together to provide assistance, support, and user-friendly programs for nurses to earn their BSN degrees (AACN, 2010; IOM, 2011).

RN Specialty Practice and Advanced Roles

Greater diversity lies in the career directions your RN license can provide. Once you finish school, you will be prepared to work as a novice nurse in many types of settings. Not all settings hire nurses right out of school, but as a new graduate, you have multiple options for employment, especially if you have flexibility in hours, shifts, and location. In a short period of time on the job, you will begin to gain expertise in certain types of nursing. For example, some nurses gain expertise in a certain age group of patients, such as pediatrics or geriatrics. Some nurses gain expertise in types of diseases, such as heart diseases, cancer, or mental health. Other nurses gain expertise in caring for patients in highly specialized settings, such as the emergency department, the operating room, or the community clinic. Still others become jack-of-all-trades by caring for many types of patients presenting with many types of health problems. My point here is that you can quickly specialize by seeking employment and opportunities in the types of nursing that interests you most. Some specialties, such as critical care, take many years to develop significant expertise; however, even as a new nurse, you can create a plan to gain knowledge and experiences that will help you establish and maintain expertise (see Chapter 9).

To help develop specialized practice, consider joining a nursing specialty organization as soon as you become a nurse. These organizations provide additional learning and development opportunities, as well as networking and leads on potential jobs. Sigma Theta Tau International (STTI), a nursing honor and scholarship society, lists over 50 organizations geared toward clinical specialties (STTI, 2011). These specialties range from neonatal nursing to hospice care nursing, literally everything from birth to death. In addition, other organizations are available to meet the needs of different groups of nurses, such as the National Black Nurses Association and the American Assembly for Men in Nursing. Still other organizations focus on various nursing roles, such as nurse educators or nurse practitioners. Some of these organizations have local chapters, making it easy to become involved. Other organizations provide opportunities on a national, or even global, level. In addition, many of these organizations serve like-minded nurses representing various nursing roles. For example, the American Association of Neuroscience Nurses meets the educational and networking needs for beginning RNs as well as advanced practice nurses.

Many nurses have rewarding careers at the bedside providing expert hands-on care to patients. But other opportunities abound for nurses by moving into advanced nursing roles. Some of these roles, such as nursing management or nursing education, have not always required education beyond a bachelor's degree. Today, more employers are requiring that these nurses obtain graduate degrees. Other advanced roles require graduate education for legal recognition. Table 1.1 provides a brief description of the more common types of advanced roles and the educational requirements for each, although other advanced roles in research, government, or health policy are available.

Many of you have heard of master's and PhD (Doctor of Philosophy) degrees. In 2006, AACN clarified another type of degree, the practice doctorate. This degree is common in many professions, yet had always been inconsistent in nursing. Although considered a *terminal degree* (highest degree) in nursing, the practice doctorate differs from the PhD. The PhD places great emphasis on research and *creating* new knowledge for the profession. This degree is well suited for preparing nurse researchers and nurse educators. The Doctor of Nursing Practice (DNP) degree has greater emphasis on the *application* of research in advanced practice. This degree is well suited for preparing advanced clinical nurses, as well as nurse educators (AACN, 2006).

TABLE 1.1   Advanced Roles in Nursing and Their Educational Requirements

ROLE	DESCRIPTION	EDUCATIONAL REQUIREMENT
Nurse Executive	Nurse executives design, facilitate, and manage patient care delivery. They are mainly involved in management and administrative issues, plan and develop procedures and policies, and handle the budgets of health care facilities, such as hospitals, nursing homes, and health clinics. (NursingSchools.com, 2012)	Bachelor's degree minimum, Master's degree or higher preferred
Nurse Educator Practice	Nurse educators are expert nurses who use evidenced-based teaching methods and learner supports to educate, counsel, advise, and prepare future nurses.	Master's degree minimum, Doctor of Nursing Practice or PhD are preferred
Clinical Nurse Leader (CNL)	The CNL designs, implements, and evaluates client care by coordinating, delegating, and supervising the care provided by the health care team, including licensed nurses, technicians, and other health professionals in all types of settings. (AACN, 2007)	Master's degree or higher
Nurse Practitioner	The NP role varies from state to state and by specialty, though the NP role generally provides primary care services. NPs may diagnose numerous conditions and prescribe various treatments and therapies. They also focus on health promotion and wellness. (American Academy of Nurse Practitioners, 2010)	Specialized Master's degree; Doctor of Nursing Practice or PhD are preferred
Clinical Nurse Specialist (CNS)	CNSs are expert clinicians in a specialized area of nursing practice. They influence care outcomes by providing expert consultation for nursing staffs and by implementing improvements in health care delivery systems. (National Association of Clinical Nurse Specialists, 2012)	Specialized Master's degree; Doctor of Nursing Practice or PhD are preferred
Nurse Midwife	Nurse midwives provide a full range of women's health services, including primary care, gynecologic and family planning services, care during pregnancy, childbirth, and care of the normal newborn. (American College of Nurse Midwives, 2010)	Specialized Master's degree; Doctor of Nursing Practice or PhD are preferred
Nurse Anesthetist (CRNA)	CRNAs provide anesthetics to patients in every practice setting, and for every type of surgery or procedure. (American Association of Nurse Anesthetists, 2012)	Specialized Master's degree; Doctor of Nursing Practice or PhD are preferred

It is the hope of AACN and other nurse leaders to require all future advanced practice nurses to earn the DNP degree in order to get their advanced nursing licenses. The IOM (2011) issued a bold recommendation that the profession double the number of nurses with doctoral degrees by 2020 in order to meet the demands of a more complicated health care system. Many schools of nursing are changing their master's degree programs to DNP programs. Current advanced practice nurses are encouraged to return to school to upgrade their education degrees.

MEN WANTED

It's no surprise to you that women dominate nursing, but it may be surprising just how underrepresented men are in nursing. The most recent data show that 7.1% of working nurses are men, and 6.6% of all nurses overall are men (USDHHS, 2010). Although these rates are up from previous years, few health professions are as gender-lopsided as is nursing. There are many reasons for the imbalance, and several chapters in this book discuss these reasons in detail. But gender imbalance is a problem since it doesn't provide diversity. The benefits of having a diverse nursing workforce that mirrors the population have been discussed for years. At the most simple level, patients may relate better to nurses who are like them—in age, race, background, and in gender. Recently, nursing and health care leaders have begun to recognize the gender imbalance as problematic. (Historically, discussions of diversity have focused only on racial and ethnic diversity.) For example, AACN (2011b) stated that "the need to attract students from underrepresented groups in nursing, specifically men…is gaining in importance…" (para. 1). They further stated "All national nursing organizations…agree that recruitment of underrepresented groups into nursing is a priority for the nursing profession in the US" (para. 8). Also, the IOM (2011) specifically noted men as underrepresented in the nursing workforce and that all groups should work together to increase workforce diversity. Unfortunately, AACN and other groups have not yet put much work or money into programs designed to bring more men into nursing, unlike resources that have been devoted to attracting other groups into nursing.

Still some efforts are underway to attract more men to nursing. Johnson and Johnson's "Dare to Care" television ad campaign has featured male nurses for several years now. Several schools are specifically targeting men to enroll or providing supports designed to meet the needs of male students. Some of these schools have been named "Best School or College of Nursing for Men" by the American Assembly for Men in Nursing (2011). It is possible that these efforts are starting to make some progress, though word-of-mouth may be having even a larger effect. According to AACN (2012b), 11.4% of BSN students, 9.9% of master's degree students, 6.8% of PhD students, and 9.4% of DNP students were male in 2011. This represents an increase from previous years. Clearly, these numbers will not fix the gender imbalance in nursing right away. Men are needed in nursing, and needed in much larger numbers. The door is open for you.

SUMMARY

In recent years, many thousands of people have lost their jobs, or have had to take cuts in pay or hours just to keep their jobs. Many others worry that their jobs may not be around in the future, or they feel that their jobs no longer fulfill or satisfy them. This is not the case with nurses. Nursing is one of the few careers that seems to weather hard economic times. Nursing continued to grow during the recent recession, and growth is expected to increase as the demand for nurses in the near future increases. This demand will provide job security and attractive salaries. Also, nurses continue to make strong and rewarding connections with their patients. These connections have earned nurses the highest levels of respect from the general public.

As health care becomes more advanced and complex, nurses' responsibilities and educational requirements have increased. This has provided challenges that nurses find stimulating and career advancement opportunities that continue to grow. With on-going learning and experience, nurses can obtain high levels of expertise. Many nurses choose to spend their careers as expert bedside nurses. Others pursue careers in administration or education. Others pursue advanced careers as high-level clinicians, researchers, and policy makers. Most of these roles require further education. Nurse leaders and the IOM are pushing for a more educated nursing workforce. Schools, employers, and institutions are working together to help nurses continue their education.

These benefits and opportunities contribute to the high levels of satisfaction nurses have about their jobs and careers. Job satisfaction contributes to a good life. It's no wonder, then, that so many young people are giving nursing a serious look. Yet today, nursing remains one of the most gender-lopsided health professions. Nurse leaders now recognize the imbalance as a problem. Men are strongly encouraged to consider a career in nursing. Clearly, there is no better time than now to be a nurse!

REFERENCES

Aiken, L. H., Clarke, S. P., Cheung, R. B., Sloane, D. M., & Silber, J. H. (2003). Educational levels of hospital nurses and surgical patient mortality. *JAMA, 290*(12), 1617–1623.

Aiken, L. H., Clarke, S. P., Sloane, D. M., Lake, E. T., & Cheney, T. (2008). Effects of hospital care environment on patient mortality and nurse outcomes. *Journal of Nursing Administration, 38*(5), 223–229.

American Academy of Nurse Practitioners. (2010). *What are nurse practitioners?* Retrieved from http://www.aanp.org/NR/rdonlyres/A1D9B4BD-AC5E-45BF-9EB0-DEFCA1123204/4710/2011FAQswhatisanNPupdated.pdf

American Assembly for Men in Nursing. (2011). *Awards: Best school/college for men in nursing.* Retrieved from http://www.aamn.org/awschool.shtml

American Association of Colleges of Nursing. (2006). *The essentials of doctoral education for advanced nursing practice.* Retrieved from http://www.aacn.nche.edu/publications/position/DNPEssentials.pdf

American Association of Colleges of Nursing. (2007). *White paper on the education and role of the clinical nurse leader.* Retrieved from http://www.aacn.nche.edu/publications/white-papers/ClinicalNurseLeader.pdf

American Association of Colleges of Nursing. (2010). *Tri-Council for Nursing issues new consensus policy statement on the educational advancement of registered nurses.* Retrieved from http://www.aacn.nche.edu/education-resources/TricouncilEdStatement.pdf

American Association of Colleges of Nursing. (2011a). *New AACN data on nursing enrollments and employment of BSN graduates.* Retrieved from http://www.aacn.nche.edu/news/articles/2011/11enrolldata

American Association of Colleges of Nursing. (2011b). *Fact sheet: Enhancing diversity in the nursing workforce.* Retrieved from http://www.aacn.nche.edu/media-relations/diversityFS.pdf

American Association of Colleges of Nursing. (2012a). *Fact sheet: The impact of education on nursing practice.* Retrieved from http://www.aacn.nche.edu/media-relations/fact-sheets/impact-of-education

American Association of Colleges of Nursing. (2012b). *New AACN data show an enrollment surge in baccalaureate and graduate programs amid calls for more highly educated nurses.* Retrieved from http://www.aacn.nche.edu/news/articles/2012/enrollment-data

American Association of Nurse Anesthetists. (2012). *Become a CRNA.* Retrieved from http://www.aana.com/ceandeducation/becomeacrna/Pages/default.aspx

American College of Nurse Midwives. (2010). *Our scope of practice.* Retrieved from http://www.midwife.org/index.asp?bid=17

Anna Maria College. (2012). *BSN degrees becoming a requirement.* Retrieved from http://www.online.annamaria.edu/hospitals-require-bsn-degrees.asp

Auerbach, D. I., Buerhaus, P. I., & Staiger, D. O. (2011). Registered nurse supply grows faster than projected amid surge in new entrants ages 23–26. *Health Affairs, 30*(12), 2286–2292.

Buerhaus, P. I., & Auerbach, D. I. (2011). The recession's effect on hospital registered nurse employment growth. *Nursing Economics, 29*(4), 163–167.

Bureau of Labor Statistics, U.S. Department of Labor. (2012a). *Occupational outlook handbook 2012–13 edition, registered nurses.* Retrieved from http://www.bls.gov/ooh/healthcare/registered-nurses.htm

Bureau of Labor Statistics, U.S. Department of Labor. (2012b). *Occupational employment and wages, May 2011: 29-1111 registered nurses.* Retrieved from http://www.bls.gov/oes/current/oes291111.htm

Dohm, A., & Shniper, L. (2007). *Occupational employment projections to 2016.* Washington, DC: US Department of Labor, Bureau of Labor Statistics.

Friese, C. R., Lake, E. T., Aiken, L. H., Silber, J. H., & Sochalski, J. (2008). Hospital nurse practice environments and outcomes for surgical oncology patients. *Health Services Research, 43*(4), 1145–1163.

Gallup. (2012). *Nurses top honesty and ethics list for 11th year.* Retrieved from http://www.gallup.com/poll/145043/nurses-top-honesty-ethics-list-11-year.aspx?version=print

Institute of Medicine. (2011). *The future of nursing: Leading change, advancing health.* Washington, DC: National Academies Press.

Kendall-Gallagher, K., Aiken, L. H., Sloane, D. M., & Cimiotti, J. P. (2011). Nurse specialty certification, inpatient mortality, and failure to rescue. *Journal of Nursing Scholarship, 43*(2), 188–194.

LPNtraining.org. (2012). *What does a licensed professional nurse do?* Retrieved from http://www.lpntraining.org/what-does-a-licensed-professional-nurse-do.html

National Association of Clinical Nurse Specialists. (2012). *CNS FAQs.* Retrieved from http://www.nacns.org/html/cns-faqs.php

NursingSchools.com. (2012). *Nurse executive*. Retrieved from http://www.nursing-schools.net/profiles/nurse-executive/

Oregon Center for Nursing. (2010). *Career satisfaction among Oregon's registered nurses: A report from the Oregon Center for Nursing*. Portland, OR: Author.

Raines, C. F., & Taglaireni, M. E. (2008, September 30). Career pathways in nursing: Entry points and academic progression. *Online Journal of Issues in Nursing, 13*(3).

Sigma Theta Tau International. (2011). *North America nursing organizations*. Retrieved from http://www.nursingsociety.org/career/careermap/pages/nursing_orgs.aspx

U.S. Department of Health and Human Services. (2010). *The registered nurse population: Findings from the 2008 National Sample Survey of Registered Nurses*. Washington, DC: U.S. Department of Health and Human Services, Health Resources and Services Administration.

TWO

Men in Nursing—It's NOT Something New!

Men have worked as nurses as far back as anyone can tell. This fact may surprise you. The growing attention the public gives to men in nursing would suggest that male nurses are a recent happening, or that men are turning to nursing only now because of recent economic troubles. It's easy to understand this confusion. Most people think that nursing started some 150 years ago with the work of Florence Nightingale. Although Nightingale's work was significant, she was not the world's first nurse. People have been sick and injured since the beginning of time. In the past, countless numbers of women *and* men have served as nurses. Unfortunately, historians have been neglectful, and perhaps even unkind, in their writings about the important role men have had in building the nursing profession.

Howard Zinn (2003) noted that historians are far from objective when they write about historical events. Presented with an infinite amount of information, historians choose what to report, emphasize, and interpret about the past. The information historians leave out of books may be just as important as what they include. In fact, the choice to exclude information may create stereotypes, myths, and cultural biases, or strengthen stereotypes that are already common. Historians often emphasize historical information that supports their own values and beliefs or that supports the beliefs that are dominant in their societies. For example, Zinn observed that most American children learn about the "settling" of North America by Europeans; however, few schoolchildren learn about the genocide of Native Americans by European settlers. Since many people never learned the *whole* story of the European colonization of North America, they are confused as to why some Native Americans protest the Columbus Day holiday. Another example is the recent criticism of Japanese schools that exclude information about the atrocities against Chinese citizens during the Japanese occupation of China during World War II.

And so it goes with nursing. Most of nursing history has been written in the last 100 years, and much of this has been written by women. It should be no surprise that most of this writing has emphasized the interests of women (Bullough, 1994). First, it is likely that some authors have emphasized the accomplishments of women in nursing as a means to inspire today's women. Second, it is likely that some authors may have wanted to balance the dominance men have in a patriarchal society (see Chapter 3). Third, some authors have reinforced the emphasis on women by retelling the history that had already been written. Regardless, most of the classic textbooks on nursing history devote very little space to men in nursing. When men have been mentioned, they are often mislabeled as administrators, soldiers, or attendants. This denies or hides their identities as nurses.

The denial of men's rightful place in nursing's history is more than just an academic concern; it denies men gender-appropriate nursing role models. This is important since role models provide us with guidance and inspiration, particularly as we take on new roles or encounter life changes. Role models give us something to aspire to. Role models of the past can teach us how men shaped the values of nursing and how they made those values come alive as they cared for their patients. Modern role models can teach us how men can apply nursing values in today's changing health care environment. Unfortunately, men have reported that the lack of role models with whom they can identify creates a sense of isolation and uncertainty as they pursue a nursing career (Kelly, Shoemaker, & Steele, 1996; O'Lynn, 2004).

The story of men's history in nursing must include accounts of individual male nurses who have contributed greatly to their patients, their communities, and the development of nursing as a whole. Men need to hear about these male role models, but so do women. The story of men's history in nursing will illuminate for women that men are not some new invaders of nursing, but rather a familiar and trusted team member. In this chapter, I will not provide a full account of men's history in nursing. Instead, I will focus on introducing you to a select group of inspirational male nurses. This chapter will follow a chronological format, starting from very early times and proceeding to the present. I will give a brief overview of what was happening in nursing during a certain period of time and then give a short account of certain male nurses from that time period. Each nurse's story will end with lessons for today's nurse. At a minimum, you should find these male nurses intriguing. I believe, however, that the work of these men will inspire you and other nurses to become today's great nurses and the role models of tomorrow.

EARLY NURSES

Men worked as nurses in ancient times, though most remain unnamed. We know very few details about early nurses, either male or female, because not much was written in those days about the work and lives of these nurses. Understanding these early nurses becomes difficult because it's not always clear who was a nurse. Our idea of a nurse as an employee or a professional is a modern concept. In early societies, there were always people who took care of others. But when does caring for others make that person a nurse? Where are the lines of distinction among early physicians, healers, shamans, and nurses? Historians have taken great liberties in addressing these uncertainties, sometimes to the detriment to the recognition of male nurses from long ago (see Chapter 3). Using a more modern perspective, taking care of a loved one at home does not make you a nurse, even though you might use nursing skills. Instead, caring for a loved one makes you a caregiver. Today, we recognize that nursing involves specialized education that allows you to take care of strangers as a means of employment. Nursing involves working for some sort of gain, whether it is financial, altruistic, or both. Nursing today does not always require working outside the home, but nursing always extends beyond the family role. This is not to say that women never provided nursing care because they were confined to staying at home. Rather, this perspective is meant to shed light on men employed throughout the centuries in a nursing role. It is this modern perspective that will frame how I identify early nurses in this chapter.

Ancient Times

The earliest records of trained individuals caring for the sick and injured were of men in ancient Greece. These men worked with Greek doctors who were probably their supervisors (Christman, 1988a; Nutting & Dock, 1935). It's not clear what these men did specifically. Possibly, these men provided hands-on care and instructed both patients and their families about their health care, just as nurses do today. We know much more about male nurses in ancient India. In the 3rd century B.C.E., King Asoka required all hospitals to follow strict guidelines for cleanliness, ventilation, and comfort. Nurses working in these hospitals were required to attend school and follow a strict moral code. Nutting and Dock (1935) reported that Lesson IX of the *Charkar-Samhita* required nurses to be intelligent, loyal, and obedient, and had to understand the connections between the mind and the body. Only men were allowed to go to nursing school and work as nurses since women were not considered worthy enough to be nurses in ancient Indian society. In school, men became skilled in cooking, bathing, massage, physical therapy, bed making, and the general care of patients. They had to know about drugs and how to prepare and administer medications. The same types of lessons were used to teach nursing students worldwide for centuries to come (Nutting & Dock, 1935).

Elsewhere, in ancient Rome, the best health care was provided to soldiers. On the battlefield, injured soldiers were cared for by other soldiers, much like they are today. However, when the soldiers returned to Roman cities, injured soldiers stayed at military hospitals called *valetudinaria*. These hospitals employed specially trained men, *nosocomi*, as nurses. *Nosocomi* were common in hospitals throughout the Roman Empire until the Middle Ages (Nutting & Dock, 1935).

The Early Christian Era

Over the next few centuries, as large numbers of people in Europe and the Middle East converted to Christianity, the Church played a larger role in the social fabric and politics of local communities. Charity and caring for one's neighbor became important values of early Christians, but these values were not often considered important by local governments in most towns and cities. Therefore, the Church usually served as the primary human and health service organization in most towns. Needy people flocked to the homes of local bishops and church members. Local churches built cloisters, covered porches, and other additions to homes and churches to house these people and provide them hospitality (food and lodging) services and nursing care. In reality, these additions to homes and churches became the first hospitals in the West serving the general public, especially the poor. At first, local church members provided the services and care in these early hospitals. As the demand for services grew, church members could not take any more time away from their families and their work, so the clergy, especially monks and some nuns, soon took over hospital services. These clergy could devote many hours of service as a way to fulfill part of their religious vows. In time, so many clergy took over nursing duties that Roman Emperor Justinian (who reigned from 527 to 565 CE) gave bishops authority over all local hospitals in the empire. Soon afterward, the number of hospitals grew, as did religious orders dedicated to caring for the sick and the poor (Nutting & Dock, 1935).

In these early years, most of the patients in hospitals were men. Men were more likely than women to leave the home for travel, work, or military pursuits. If they took ill, they could not be cared for by family members because they were too far from home. These men would go to hospitals and receive their care from local male nurses. Early hospitals employed many male nurses, since it was improper for women to provide personal care to male strangers, just as it was improper for men to care for women. This taboo persisted until the early 20th century, and is still common in more traditional societies today.

Also, during these times, women's health care was not seen as very important. If women became sick, they had to rely on family members or neighbors for care, although many women used the services of midwives for their medical care. If no one was available to tend to their needs, women often went to convents for nursing care from nuns (Nutting & Dock, 1935). Over the centuries, more hospitals were able to care for female patients by eventually using female nurses.

The clergy also used the services of groups of men known as *parabolani*. These men were responsible for seeking out the sick and bringing them to the hospital. Some of these men may have worked like today's home health nurses, giving simple care services in the home and referring patients to hospitals if necessary. These men provided a valuable service, since the public feared many illnesses such as the plague. Out of fear, families often abandoned their loved ones who came down with some unusual or disfiguring disease. Without these men, many people would have simply died in the streets or in make-shift shelters. Some authors have praised the work of the *parabolani* (Donahue, 1996; Mellish, 1990); however Nutting and Dock (1935) had a more cautious view. They reported that since illness was often feared, the work of the *parabolani* was dangerous. It was difficult to find men who would do this kind of nursing work. Low-level monks and unemployed men were often forced into these jobs. In many cities, the *parabolani* became notorious for their meanness and illegal activities, such as taking bribes. The behaviors became so bad that many bishops disbanded these groups by the middle of the 5th century (Nutting & Dock, 1935). By this time, church members and other religious groups took over home care and the care of those who had been abandoned by others.

Role Model: St. Basil the Great

St. Basil the Great was born around 329 CE in what is now Turkey. When his father died, Basil was sent to school for a religious education in nearby Caesarea and later in Athens. He returned to Caesarea and was baptized by the local bishop. He devoted all his energy to religious studies and eventually started a monastery near his family's home. In 363 CE, he became a priest and took a position in the administrative work of the diocese. He was known as a wise and just administrator who often stood up for the poor. The historical record is not clear about his nursing work at this point; however, it is likely that he provided hands-on care to those in need during his religious training and early priesthood. Writings about St. Basil do suggest that he served the poor, provided hospitality to strangers, and cared for the needs of the hungry during times of famine (McSorely, 1907). He may have functioned like today's community/population health nurses by assessing the needs of the poor and mobilizing resources to fill those needs. Basil became the Bishop of Caesarea in 370 CE and served as bishop until his death in 379 CE.

In his teachings, St. Basil scolded the wealthy for not helping those in need. In response to the lavish homes of the rich, St. Basil used Church resources to build a large and magnificent complex called *Ptochoptopheion* in the middle of the wealthiest suburb of Caesarea. The complex was so large that it practically became its own city and was called "Newtown" and "City of Mercy." At Newtown, Basil and his workers cared for strangers, the sick, and the homeless, and gave job training to those without marketable skills. Since the hospital was located next to the luxurious homes of the rich, Newtown became a constant reminder to the wealthy of their obligation to help the poor. Newtown quickly became the best hospital in the Western world. Others used Newtown as a model for future hospitals, including the hospitals built later in Constantinople and Alexandria (McSorely, 1907; Nutting & Dock, 1935).

Lessons for today's nurse

St. Basil the Great was an advocate for vulnerable people. I define *advocacy* as standing up for and giving voice to people who cannot do it for themselves. Advocates may face an uphill battle, may go against the opinions of others, or even put themselves in risk for the benefit of others. Even though St. Basil was a powerful bishop, his actions opposed the wealthy and other bishops of his time. St. Basil used his passions, talents, and local influence to direct resources in order to build a large and famous hospital. Newtown helped the people and visitors of Caesarea, but also Newton inspired hospitals and service to the sick and poor across the Western world. St. Basil was tenacious in his assault on the greed and self-serving lives of the wealthy of his day. He provides an early example of how to translate personal values into actions that improve the quality of health care.

THE MIDDLE AGES AND THE RENAISSANCE

Early hospitals flourished in the years after St. Basil established Newtown. Many of the hospitals in Western Europe remained small and served a local population and visitors. Some of these hospitals provided short-term hospitality services only; others provided a full array of health and human services. Nurses working in these hospitals were often monks or other religious persons tied to the local church or monastery. Other hospitals opened in Eastern Europe and the Middle East as well (Lascaratos, Kalantzis, & Poulakou-Rebelakou, 2004). Many of these hospitals were established by emperors, noblemen, bishops, and the wealthy as demonstrations of their religious values of charity. Soon, homes designed to care for the elderly began to appear. These facilities, called *gerocomeia* (Greek for "elderly care"), were often built near monasteries or existing hospitals. These homes were unusual since, in those times, families usually took care of their older relatives. But not all of the elderly had family who could or would care for them. One of these homes, built in Constantinople, could house 24 residents and was staffed by six male nurses. These men provided daily care for the residents. If the residents became ill, the nurses would take them to the nearby hospital (Lascaratos et al., 2004).

The Military Religious Orders

As the first millennium approached, many Christians believed that the Apocalypse was close at hand. Increasing numbers of European Christians began making pilgrimages to the Holy Land to pray for their salvation. Hostels were established as early as 603 CE in Jerusalem to provide food and shelter to these pilgrims (Sire, 1994). These hostels were necessary since a trip to the Holy Land was exhausting, time-consuming, and dangerous. Many pilgrims took ill along the way or were victims of thieves and other criminals. Pilgrims often arrived in need of medical care, so the need for hospitals grew. At about the same time, the first wave of Crusaders arrived in efforts to take the Holy Land away from local Moslem rulers. Military religious orders (organizations) were formed to organize the Crusaders. These military orders also opened hospitals and cared for the injured and sick, which is why these orders were sometimes called "hospitaller" orders. Most of these hospitals cared for wounded soldiers, but they also cared for local residents too.

Most historians acknowledged that men worked as nurses in these military orders, but many of them got it wrong by oversimplifying the structure and work of the military orders (e.g., Bainbridge, 2001; Donahue, 1996; Mellish, 1990). This error has reduced the importance of men's true place in nursing's history. Typically, authors described the members of these military orders as soldiers who served as nurses only because it was necessary. But most orders had members whose primary duty was to serve as nurses and who only served as soldiers when absolutely necessary. The regular soldiers helped the nurses when they were not in battle (Nutting & Dock, 1935; Sire, 1994).

Three major military orders operated hospitals in the Holy Land during the Crusades: the Knights Hospitallers of St. John of Jerusalem (now the

Sovereign Military Order of Malta, or the Knights of Malta), the Knights of St. Lazarus, and the Teutonic Knights (Nutting & Dock, 1935). Each order operated differently in their military pursuits as well as in how they ran their hospitals. For example, the Knights of St. Lazarus in Jerusalem focused on caring for lepers (Sire, 1994). The Teutonic Knights assumed both military and hospital functions when they started, whereas the Knights of Malta formed a hospital first and then took on a military role only after the Crusades were underway (Nutting & Dock, 1935). In time, the battles intensified. Most of the orders had to increase the number of soldiers, but this was not enough to keep the Holy Land in the Crusaders' hands. When the Europeans were eventually driven out of the Holy Land, the military orders focused on internal struggles and conquests in Europe. Their focus on caring for the sick diminished, except for the Knights of Malta (Sire, 1994). Of these three military orders, only the Knights of Malta survives today. Its founder, Brother Gerard, serves as an ideal role model from the religious military orders.

Role Model: Brother Gerard

Although we know little about the details of Brother Gerard's life, he is given credit for founding the Hospitallers of St. John (Knights of Malta), an organization with a long history of men serving as nurses. The Knights of Malta were probably the first military order in the Holy Land, predating the Crusades by some 50 years. By the mid-11th century, Moslem rulers were relatively welcoming to the growing number of Christians making pilgrimages to the Holy Land. In order to meet the religious needs of pilgrims, but also sensing economic opportunities in the Holy Land, wealthy merchants from the Italian city of Amalfi established a Benedictine abbey in Jerusalem named St. Mary of the Latins. By 1080, the abbey had built a large hospital to handle the lodging, food, and health care needs of large numbers of pilgrims coming to the city. The hospital was built on the site where it is believed an angel arrived to announce the birth of St. John the Baptist, so it was called the Hospital of St. John (Sire, 1994).

Before long, the Benedictine monks could not keep up with the demands for services. Instead of limiting the number of people who could stay at the hospital, Brother Gerard devised a new system of staffing the hospital. At that time, most hospitals were staffed by monks and other clergy. Brother Gerard invited lay persons (people who were not part of the clergy) to devote their lives to religious service but without taking the religious vows of clergy or living secluded lives in monasteries. Brother Gerard believed that people could serve God more effectively with hands-on acts of mercy rather than all-day prayer (Sire, 1994). Acting on this belief, Brother Gerard created a system of lay service that is common in many faith communities today. His changes increased the number of men who could work as nurses.

As the hospital was being built, the fighting among feudal lords, rulers, and kings became so intense that it threatened to jeopardize the stability of Europe. With so much internal fighting, Europe would be less able to protect itself from the advancing armies from Moslem and Asian kingdoms. Fearing the destruction of a Christian Europe, and possibly eyeing economic opportunities of controlling the Middle East, Pope Urban II made a plea to powerful and wealthy men, knights, and warriors to unite against a common enemy—Moslem rulers in the Holy Land. In 1095, the Pope authorized the first Crusade, and soon warriors stormed into Jerusalem and surrounding cities. Brother Gerard's Hospital of St. John became a staging area for the soldiers, a place of refuge, a center for procuring supplies for the armies, and a place to treat and nourish injured and sick soldiers. The abbey monks probably tended to the spiritual needs of soldiers too (Sire, 1994).

The first Crusade was very successful for the Europeans. They quickly took control of the Holy Land from local rulers. Many of the Crusaders were grateful to Brother Gerard for his support. The soldiers donated portions of their wealth and newly conquered territories to the hospital. However, instead of corrupting himself with these lavish donations, Brother Gerard used this wealth to build seven other hospitals throughout the Holy Land. He also convinced a number of soldiers to stay behind and serve a religious life as nurses in these hospitals. Other soldiers stayed to provide security services and protect pilgrims from bandits and other criminals. By 1113, Brother Gerard's organization had grown so large that Pope Paschal II incorporated Brother Gerard's group into a religious military order. This made the Knights of Malta the first great military order of the Middle Ages (Sire, 1994).

Brother Gerard was the first leader to combine the religious value of altruism (the unselfish devotion to the welfare of others) with chivalry values of commitment and loyal service to one's lord or leader. Brother Gerard taught his followers to consider poor and travel-weary pilgrims as their lords. Followers were expected to serve the poor with the commitment and fervor expected of a knight who serves his king. With more travelers arriving in Jerusalem who were injured or ill, Brother Gerard's followers also devoted themselves to nursing. Brother Gerard's call to serve the sick and poor became the central focus of the Knights of Malta. Shortly after his death in 1120, these values were adopted into the official rules of the Order (Sire, 1994).

Lessons for today's nurse

Brother Gerard's beliefs about expanding acts of service to God beyond the walls of a church or monastery and into the hospital were revolutionary. He seized the opportunity to infuse his religious values into the chivalry code that was popular and powerful at that time. The lesson we learn here is that personal values, no matter how altruistic, are of little benefit unless they are activated into direct service. In other words, it's not enough to want, hope, and pray for the relief of suffering. As individuals, we must roll up our sleeves and display our values by providing direct assistance to those in need. Brother Gerard used the cultural codes of chivalry already in use by knights and soldiers to attract men to join him in his work in a way that created commitment to service to others. As nurses we must do the same. We must examine the cultural beliefs and practices that are present in our communities and use them as vehicles to display the nursing values of care and comfort (Leininger, 1991). By doing this, we will gain the respect of those we serve and motivate others to serve the needs of their own communities.

The Nonmilitary Religious Nursing Orders

Nurse historians give little attention to the many nonmilitary religious orders that sprang up in Europe during and after the Crusades.For example, Gaston of Dauphine founded the Hospital Brothers of St. Anthony in 1095. The men of this order specialized in caring for people suffering from bacterial infections of the skin, otherwise known as St. Anthony's Fire. Over the next 700 years, the Brothers built and served in hospitals throughout Europe until they eventually merged with the Knights of Malta (Rudge, 1907; Sire, 1994). Another group, the Alexian Brothers, trace their roots to a group of people called *beguines*, who cared for the sick and dying as early as 1057 (Alexian Brothers, 2005; Tranbarger, 2007a). A subgroup of the Alexian Brothers in Germany focused their mission on burying those who died from the plague, since no one else would bury the corpses out of fear of catching the plague. The Alexian Brothers eventually expanded their mission to providing nursing care for the sick in their homes. They established their expertise in public health and psychiatric care. They built and operated hospitals throughout Europe. They even came to the United States, where they built nursing schools for men. They are still active today in Europe and the United States, where they operate a number of health care organizations and continue to work as nurses. These groups, along with other religious orders that did not have a military component, had more visibility and influence in their local communities than did the military nursing orders established during the Crusades.

Role Model: St. Camillus de Lellis

Camillus was born in Italy in a noble family in 1550, where he lived an early life of wealth and self-indulgence. At 17, he joined the army, where he developed a reputation for having a violent temper and being a troublemaker. The army discharged him dishonorably after four years. Camillus became a chronic gambler and wandered the countryside penniless. When his father died, Camillus yearned to turn his life around. He became friends with a Franciscan monk who convinced Camillus to join the Franciscans. Camillus spent time with the Franciscans, but they would not accept him as a member because he had a chronic and infected wound on his leg (Campbell, 1908; Monk, 1984; O'Connell-Cahill, 1991).

Camillus went to the hospital of San Giacomo in Rome to offer his employment in exchange for medical care. They agreed to take him, but he was soon fired due to his bad temper. He returned to his gambling habit and troubled ways. Eventually, he tried to go back to the Franciscans, but again, they would not admit him because of his leg, which had grown much worse. Camillus went back to the hospital, but this time, he was confined to bed. His confinement, along with spiritual counseling, taught Camillus patience. He used his suffering and pain as a means to grow spiritually. His wound improved in time, so Camillus began to work as a nurse to pay off his debt. The old Camillus disappeared. The hospital grew to love the piety and prudence he displayed. In time, he was made superintendent of the hospital (Campbell, 1908; Monk, 1984; O'Connell-Cahill, 1991).

The indifference and lack of compassion displayed by many of the hospital nurses bothered Camillus. Camillus vowed to be a different kind of nurse. Goodier (1959) noted that

> [h]e began to love the patients in the hospital, not merely to serve them; and the more he loved them, the more he was troubled by the treatment they received, even in a well-regulated hospital like San Giacomo. One evening…the thought occurred to him that good nursing depended on love and [how much better it would be] independent of wages. If he could gather men about him who would nurse for love…then he might raise nursing to the standard he desired. (para. 36)

Camillus gathered a group of like-minded men and tried to form a lay organization for male nurses, but the local bishop did not support this. He told Camillus to become a priest instead. Camillus consented, and after studying for a few years, he was ordained. As a priest, he was now free to form his nursing order. Against the advice of his spiritual mentor, Camillus set up his congregation house and hospital in the roughest neighborhood in Rome in 1586. Camillus was firm on this location since this neighborhood was where the greatest need was to be found. Camillus and his followers cared for as many patients as they could (Campbell, 1908; Goodier, 1959; Monk, 1984; O'Connell-Cahill, 1991).

Camillus realized that some of the patients who needed him the most were so sick that they couldn't leave their homes. Camillus and his followers then started to go to the homes of the sick and dying to give them the nursing care that they needed. This became the first formal home hospice service in Rome. His congregation was called the Brothers of a Happy Death since they brought such compassion and comfort to those who were dying. But this work was difficult, and his followers took great risk. In fact, two of Camillus's followers came down with the plague and died after nursing the sick who were quarantined on a ship in Naples. Despite this risk, their work was important. Many feared those who were dying and left them to care for themselves. Camillus and his followers served these dying people without question. They also travelled to battlefields to nurse the wounded and provide nursing care to prisoners (Campbell, 1908; Goodier, 1959; Monk, 1984; O'Connell-Cahill, 1991). In 1591, the Pope elevated the congregation of Camillus to a religious order. The group was given the symbol of a red cross to wear on their coats so that they could easily be recognized on the battlefields and in the streets. This symbol has since become an international symbol for health care.

Camillus served as leader and spiritual guide for the order until his own health began to fail in 1607. His chronic leg disease worsened, which made walking very difficult. However, poor health did not prevent him from his nursing passion. Camillus was known to drag himself from his sick bed to visit patients and give them care (Campbell, 1908; Goodier, 1959; Monk, 1984; O'Connell-Cahill, 1991). He died in 1614, but his worked lives on. Today, the order is known as the Order of St. Camillus Servants of the Sick.

The order operates health care facilities and human service organizations in over 35 countries (Order of St. Camillus Servants of the Sick, 2010).

Lessons for today's nurse

Clearly, St. Camillus sacrificed a great deal to care for the sick and poor. Most of us are unwilling to sacrifice everything to work as nurses. Perhaps that's why he was made a saint. There are two important lessons, however, that modern men can learn from St. Camillus. First, it's never too late to turn one's life around and help others in need. Each of us must face the consequences of any poor choices we make, especially those we make when we are young. Each of us takes a different journey in learning how our skills and talents can be used to help others. At age 24, St. Camillus had already experienced many life failures. His first attempt at nursing also failed, but he persisted even though his journey was difficult. Today, many men come to nursing after much soul-searching or after careers that have left them empty. Other men come to nursing after losing jobs they had for many years. Men of all ages and backgrounds can find much satisfaction in nursing and contribute greatly to those in need.

Second, St. Camillus teaches us that we must think of nursing, at least in part, as a *vocation*. Vocation can be defined as having a calling to a certain type of work. To have a vocation encourages you to become engaged in work that benefits others. With vocation, your values and morals become the primary reasons to select an occupation, not money. White (2002) describes vocation in nursing as being "dedicated and committed to assisting another who is disadvantaged" (p. 283). Vocation in nursing involves doing whatever is necessary and possible for the benefit of the patient.

Today, an emphasis on vocation in nursing is seen as rather controversial (White, 2002; Yam, 2004). Some authors have stated that nursing as a vocation emphasizes traditional feminine values and self-sacrifice. Vocation puts nurses in a vulnerable position, in which their devotion blinds them to systemic abuse and sets them up to be taken advantage of by supervisors, physicians, and the general public. Some have argued that vocation in nursing encourages nurses to accept long work hours, unsafe working conditions, low wages, and few opportunities for career advancement. Modern nurse leaders have fought many battles that now allow nurses to earn a fair wage and to have a powerful voice in health care. For the most part, these advances have allowed nurses to improve their ability to care for others; therefore, these efforts have been good for nurses and patients. Some have concluded that vocation in nursing will turn the clock back.

However, I disagree with vocation critics. I believe that it is possible to combine vocation in nursing without harmful self-sacrifice. Too much self-sacrifice only makes a nurse exhausted. White (2002) stated, "The good [of the patient] cannot be guaranteed by self-sacrificing behavior; it can be guaranteed only by caring for them out of a deep sense of commitment for their welfare" (p. 287). I worry, instead, about a movement away from a vocation perspective. If taken to the extreme, an exclusive view that nursing is a career will promote an "*it's all about me*," attitude when nursing should really be "*all about the patient*." When nursing turns into something that emphasizes the self-interest of the individual nurse, then we will create the types of nurse that St. Camillus criticized. Unfortunately, I have seen these nurses—nurses who sometimes put their own wants above the needs of their patients. This type of nurse gives substandard care. St. Camillus teaches us that nursing is a gift to ourselves and to our patients. Nursing, as vocation, guides us to care deeply for our patients and keep them in the center of our work. Nursing, as vocation, guides us to focus our work on comforting those in need. When we do nursing as vocation, we inspire ourselves and those around us.

THE DARK AGES OF NURSING AND THE DEMISE OF MEN IN NURSING

Mellish (1990) referred to the period between 1500 to 1800 as the Dark Ages of Nursing. Unlike the field of medicine, which advanced with growing scientific knowledge, nursing stagnated during this time. In many countries, nurses gave only low-quality custodial care. Hospital conditions became so bad that many people hired doctors and better quality nurses to care for them at home. Many hospitals became a place of last resort.

Florence Nightingale, an upper-class woman in Victorian England, was appalled by the horrible condition of London's hospitals. Against the will of her parents, she trained to become a nurse in Germany and gained fame by improving the care given to soldiers wounded in the Crimean War. After the war, she returned to England and used her knowledge, leadership, and political savvy to usher in many reforms that improved the conditions in hospitals dramatically. Her work reversed decades of neglect and apathy, and brought nursing to the beginning of its modern professionalism (Barnham, 2002). Although Nightingale did much to rescue nursing, some authors have blamed Nightingale's reforms for the literal demise of men in nursing, a process in which the number of men working as nurses in Europe and North America dropped greatly (Bartfay, 1996; Christman, 1988a; Evans, 2004; Mackintosh, 1997; Villeneuve, 1994). The reasons for the demise of men in nursing, however, are more complex than just Nightingale's reforms. Other things were underway before Nightingale's time that discouraged men from becoming nurses.

Much social and political change swept across Europe between 1500 and 1800. In many countries, the Protestant Reformation led to the closing of Catholic churches, monasteries, and convents. Hospitals run by the Catholic Church and staffed by Catholic nurses were either closed or taken over by local governments or private businesses. As Catholic nurses were driven out, they took their nursing knowledge and altruism with them. Without the financial backing of the Catholic Church, many hospitals were forced to survive on meager funds from the government or adopt a business/profit-making model. In order to make a profit, many hospitals hired untrained nurses who could be paid low wages. The lowest wages could be given to women who were social misfits, alcoholics, or prisoners, so many of these women were hired to work as nurses. Nursing soon became a very low-status occupation (Donahue, 1996; Dossey, 1999; Mackintosh, 1997; Mellish, 1990). With low wages and low status, men were not attracted to nursing work.

Catholic hospitals did survive in areas in which the population remained largely Catholic (such as France and Italy) or in areas that tolerated Catholic hospitals. However, the number of men working as nurses in these Catholic hospitals began to decline. Fewer men were entering monasteries or lay religious orders. Some lay orders of male nurses that had formed in the past started to collapse due to political infighting and lack of financial support. Others were banned by governments that were suspicious of the Catholic Church (Alexian Brothers, 2005; Moeller, 1910; Rudge, 1907). At the same time, the number of convents grew. More women entered convents and were assigned hospital service. Eventually, some Catholic hospitals preferred nuns over men to work as nurses, consistent with the male-dominated attitudes of the Church and society. In France, the large Maisons-Dieu hospitals requested only nuns, and they used male nurses only to provide personal care to men or to subdue aggressive or mentally ill patients (Nutting & Dock, 1935). Increasingly, these men functioned more as attendants than as nurses.

Also during this period, the Industrial Revolution began to take hold. Factories and industries that extracted the natural resources needed for manufactured goods sprang up across Europe and North America. Workers were needed for the mines, forests, factories, and commerce industries such as warehousing and shipping. These jobs required physical strength and long working hours away from home—requirements suitable for only men at that time. Since wages in these new industries were better than in other types of employment, men flocked to these industries and away from low-paying and low-status nursing jobs (Christman, 1988a; Donahue, 1996; Mackintosh, 1997). The takeover of hospitals by business, the increasing low status and low pay for nurses, the increased use of nuns, and the economic opportunities available for men in industry all combined to reduce the number of men working as nurses before Nightingale's reforms. Nevertheless, Nightingale's reforms created a nursing environment that drove even more men away from nursing. In fact, the remnants of her reforms continue to create an unwelcoming barrier for the large-scale return of men to the nursing profession.

Nightingale was born into an upper-class family in England in 1820. Intelligent, passionate, and dissatisfied with the unfulfilling role Victorian society had for women, Nightingale rebelled against her parents and went to Germany to become a nurse. As a nurse, she went to the battlefield hospitals of the Crimea in 1854. There, she became famous for improving the squalid conditions of the hospitals. With improved sanitation and nursing care, she saved the lives of many injured soldiers. She earned much admiration and respect back home, and a fund was started for her to open a nursing school at St. Thomas Hospital in London.

Nightingale noticed that the physicians and hospital administrators who had allowed the poor conditions to develop in English hospitals were almost exclusively men. She believed that women possessed a natural ability for caring and would do better than men in operating the hospitals. Nightingale advocated for the removal of men from organizing, supervising, and performing care services for the sick (Donahue, 1996; Dossey, 1999). She wrote in a letter in 1867 that

> [t]he whole reform in nursing both at home and abroad has consisted of this: to take all power over nursing out of the hands of men, and put it into the hands of one female trained head and make her responsible for everything. (Dossey, 1999, p. 291)

Physicians and administrators were not used to women and nurses who resisted and challenged their authority. Some hospitals refused to hire Nightingale or the nurses trained in her school. In time, however, the benefits of having trained nurses became obvious. Patients did much better and hospitals ran more smoothly under the direction of these new nurses. New schools sprang up throughout the English-speaking world to prepare more trained nurses. These new schools initially followed Nightingale's model in admitting only women. As more women became trained nurses, men could not compete for nursing positions since men could not obtain a nursing education. Over time, most men were removed from nursing positions and hired only as orderlies and attendants (Dossey, 1999; Kalisch & Kalisch, 1986). Still, a few general hospitals provided separate nursing schools for men, since men were still needed for physically aggressive patients and male patients with urologic disorders, or to care for sick male patients in their homes. Other schools for men opened in psychiatric hospitals (Crummer, 1924; Mackintosh, 1997; Tranbarger, 2007a), but schools for men were rare.

Role Model: Walt Whitman

Little is written about male nurses in the decades leading up to Nightingale's reforms. In the United States, men gave nursing care when necessary, but it is likely that few men worked as nurses full-time. For example, Sabin (1997) noted that epidemics swept the South frequently during the 19th century. During these epidemics, women and children were sent out of the cities while men stayed behind to nurse the sick. Some of these men worked like private-duty nurses, taking care of people or family members in their homes. Other men worked like traditional nurses in hospitals and shelters. Many male nurses were African American, since slaves were not allowed to leave the cities. Many slaves, both male and female, took care of White residents who were sick. Once the epidemic had passed, these temporary male nurses returned to their previous jobs and ways of life (Sabin, 1997). Other men served as nurses in battlefield hospitals during the Civil War.

Perhaps no other man working as a nurse during this period is as famous as Walt Whitman. Whitman treated the wounds of soldiers and did other tasks of the nurses, but this famous poet described himself only as a visitor and consoler to the injured soldiers in the hospitals (Roper, 2008). In effect, Whitman was one of these temporary nurses. Nevertheless, Whitman did much to make the public aware of the desperate need for nurses and the need for improved hospital conditions.

Shortly after the Civil War broke out in 1861, Whitman's brother joined the Union Army and was injured at the Battle of Fredericksburg in 1862. Whitman left home to visit his injured brother. It was near the battlefield that Whitman first experienced the army hospital. Whitman saw heaps of dead bodies and piles of amputated arms, hands, and legs. The filth of the hospitals and the desperate condition of the patients left a life-long impact on him. He moved to Washington, DC, and continued to visit injured soldiers in the hospitals for the next several years. In 1863, Whitman visited the hospitals nearly every day. He claimed to have made over 600 hospital visits and tended to 80,000–100,000 patients (Kummings, 2006; Roper, 2008).

Most of the soldiers did not know Whitman as a famous poet. Most of them were young men, who could not read. If they could read, they rarely read poetry books. Most soldiers came to know Whitman simply as a kindly gentleman, not as a celebrity who visited them only to boost his image in the eyes of the public. Whitman's visits usually included coming to a soldier's bedside to provide emotional support. Typically, Whitman took the hand of each soldier and asked how he was doing. Whitman listened to the soldier's stories, wrote letters to their families, and read to them. Whitman joked with them and helped them forget their troubles. Visits included hands-on work also. Whitman tended to the soldier's hygiene needs, fed those who could not eat, changed their dressings, and helped the physicians and nurses with procedures such as surgeries and amputations (Kummings, 2006; Roper, 2008). This work made Whitman a true nurse, not just a friendly visitor.

The hospitals employed a few regular nurses; most of them were female. Volunteers were needed to help provide care for the patients, since there was only one nurse for as many as 60 patients. Some of these female nurses kept diaries or wrote memoirs about their work in the army hospitals. In these diaries, we learn that some of the nurses did not like Whitman or his visits. The nurses enforced strict rules that Whitman often broke. For example, some of the nurses would not allow men to leave their beds and visit with other patients. Sometimes, Whitman gathered soldiers together for visits, or if they were too sick, Whitman delivered messages from one patient to another. Unlike many visitors who brought Bibles for the patients to read, Whitman brought the funny papers. Whitman came to the hospitals with a bag filled with oranges, tobacco, and stationery to give to the soldiers. Often, Whitman brought brandy and other alcoholic drinks that were forbidden by the nurses. Whitman would sneak the brandy to the patients when the nurses weren't looking or when the patients got up to use the latrine. Worst of all, Whitman usually stayed past visiting hours. The nurses retired at 8:30 pm and would leave the care of the patients to night watchmen. Whitman would stay late into the night talking with the patients, helping them write letters, and tending to their needs (Roper, 2008).

Whitman wrote a number of poems and essays about the war and the plight of soldiers in the army hospitals. The most famous collection of these poems, *Drum-Taps*, chronicles the suffering the soldiers experienced. One poem in this collection, *The Wound Dresser*, gives a powerful description of nursing work in these hospitals. The poem tells the story of the nurse going from bed to bed, tending bloody wounds and amputations, all the while trying to push away his own fatigue and sorrow (Roper, 2008). This poem became famous among nurses since it captured the reality of wartime nursing better than any other written work at that time.

Lessons for today's nurse

Although Whitman may not have been an employed nurse, he teaches us the lesson of what is now called *client-centered care*. This type of care places importance on what the patient wants and the patient's own ideas of what he or she needs, even if those wants and needs go against what nurses and physicians think is best. Client-centered care is a modern idea in nursing. It wasn't that long ago that the saying, "Doctor knows best" was used by nurses to force patients to conform to the physician's wishes. Nurses were the enforcers of the rules. (Unfortunately, some nurses still behave this way today!) Now, nurses are taught to get to know their patients, to find out their preferences and their needs, and to do what they can to mobilize resources to meet those needs. In order to do this, nurses must really listen to their patients and design their care for each patient individually.

In Whitman's day, nurses often treated patients as objects. Whitman ignored this idea. He treated each soldier with respect. He asked them to tell him stories about their lives and their experiences. He listened to them. He connected with them. He became a trusted friend whom the soldiers loved. He got to see the soldiers' worlds through their eyes. In short, Whitman got to know the patients in ways the nurses of his time almost never did. A nurse's ability to *know the patient* was something described by nurse scholars such as Christine Tanner and others over 100 years later. We now understand that knowing the patient is something nurses need to do in order to provide the care we now expect of nurses.

Whitman teaches us that nurses cannot simply give care *to* patients. Instead, nurses must care *for* patients. Caring for patients requires that we accept patients where they are in their lives, listen to their needs, and shape our care so that it fits each patient perfectly. Whitman teaches us that a simple grasp of a patient's hand is the first step in making a connection with a patient. Asking a patient how she or he is doing and really listening to what he or she has to say helps us create a type of bond with patients called *presence*. Presence builds trust and connects hearts. Whitman did not have formal training as a nurse and did not follow the practices of the nurses of his day. Instead, Whitman used his humanity, his natural heart to connect with patients. Whitman gave client-centered care simply by his desire to care for those in need.

THE 20TH CENTURY

The demise of men in nursing worsened further in the 20th century. In the early 1900s, registration laws appeared in many countries, including England, Canada, and the United States. These laws were designed to protect the public against people who claimed to be nurses, but who had no formal nursing education. In order to be eligible for registration, a nurse had to meet certain criteria, including graduation from a school of nursing approved by the government. At first, these laws barred men from joining the registration roles as full members or required men to be listed in a separate but unequal registration list. This put men at a disadvantage when people wanted to hire a private duty nurse or when hospitals verified the credentials of those applying for nursing positions (Kalisch & Kalish, 2004; Mackintosh, 1997). With difficulty finding jobs, some men left nursing for other opportunities.

Also, female nurses adopted the view that men should not be nurses. Female nurses grew more hostile to the men within their ranks in order to drive them out or prevent more men from becoming nurses. Some female nurses perpetuated negative stereotypes about male nurses and created system barriers for men in nursing. For example, men were not allowed to join the American Nurses Association (ANA) until 1930 (R. Barry, ANA librarian, personal communication, June 21, 2005), even though membership in this organization was seen as an important step for professional development. Men were denied promotions and were prevented from opportunities in the United States and in other countries.

Negative stereotypes also led to barriers for male nurses in the military, especially in the United States. During the Spanish-American War, there was a severe shortage of nurses to care for sick and injured soldiers. The military hired both male and female nurses to care for the soldiers, including female nurses who had been trained in newly formed nursing schools. The care given by the trained nurses was admired by soldiers and officers, and likely saved countless lives. After the war, Surgeon General George Miller Sternberg was opposed to keeping female nurses in the military because he felt that the male medics would be distracted if they had to work beside women. However, influential surgeons and female nurse leaders petitioned Congress to establish a female-only Army Nurse Corps in 1901 and Navy Nurse Corps in 1908 (Kalish & Kalish, 1986). Men, they believed, would make better soldiers than nurses. With the formation of these nurse corps, men were no longer allowed to serve as nurses. Due to this change, the small numbers of men enrolled in nursing school were no longer eligible to be excused from the draft even though male college students with other college majors *were* eligible. As a result, some nursing schools would not admit men because they could be drafted into the army at any time (Craig, 1956). Male enrollment in nursing schools dropped even further in the years leading up to World War II. Only 922 men graduated from nursing school between 1939 and 1940, about 1.6% of all nursing school graduates (Craig, 1940).

Just prior to World War II, the military experienced another severe shortage of nurses and was considering drafting civilian female nurses into the nurse corps. In 1940, the Men's Nurses Section of the ANA formed and immediately began asking the ANA to lobby Congress to drop the ban on men serving as nurses in the military (Men Nurses and the Armed Services, 1943; Nursing in a Democracy, 1940). By this time, the ANA had become more supportive of male nurses. In 1941, before the bombing of Pearl Harbor, the ANA sent a letter to the Surgeon General asking him to allow men to work as nurses in the military. A representative from the Surgeon General's office denied the request, noting that the country was not at war (yet) and that the employment of male nurses would be impractical. At the ANA Biennial meeting in 1942, with the country now at war, the ANA House of Delegates passed a resolution to demand that the ban be struck down. Again, the War Department and Surgeon General's office upheld the ban and requested that male nurses sign up for other health care duties, such as corpsmen, lab technicians, pharmacy technicians, and nursing assistants. Leroy Craig, Chairman of the Men's Nurses Section, stated that this was unacceptable since the military was in great need of the professional nursing services male nurses could offer (Men Nurses and the Armed Services, 1943).

Christman (1988b) noted that many male nurses wanted to serve but were not allowed to serve as nurses. Approximately 1,200 male nurses were drafted during World War II, but none could work as nurses. Other male nurses enlisted as soldiers during the war. One nurse, Jacob Rose, wrote that he was not allowed to work as a nurse, but instead, was assigned to guard empty land in Texas, fill potholes in roads in India, and clear land for a baseball field (Rose, 1947). Even worse, these male nurses were not allowed to work as medics and corpsmen "because to do so they had to go to corps school, but they were too qualified to enter that training [since they were already nurses], so they were assigned duties outside of health care" (Christman, 1988b, p. 46).

As the war progressed and eventually ended, pressure mounted to allow men to serve as nurses in the military. Between 1944 and 1955, 11 bills were introduced in Congress to strike down the military's ban (Craig, 1956). Due to unsupportive attitudes that many female nurses still held, opposition to these bills came from female nurse leaders in the Army Nurse Corps. Bester (2007) noted that Army Nurse Corps Chief Colonel Mary G. Phillips sent out a letter to senior nursing officers requesting their opinions about a bill to drop the male ban. She received the following responses:

> Nursing the sick is definitely a woman's prerogative and even though the majority of patients in the Army are men, women nurses are more acceptable and adaptable from the professional and also personal angle.
>> LTC Elsie Schneider, Letterman General Hospital,
>> San Francisco, CA; copy of letter dated January 26, 1950,
>> provided by C. Scott, May 13, 2005

> It is my opinion, therefore, that it would be extremely unwise to open the Nursing Corps to men nurses at this time.
>> LTC Ida Danielson, Army Medical Center, Washington, DC;
>> copy of letter dated January 18, 1950,
>> provided by C. Scott, May 13, 2005

> Personally, I prefer that we do not have male nurses, but if Congress authorizes their admission, I hope that the number allotted in the Corps will be in proportion to the entire civilian registered nurse population.
>> LTC Elizabeth Fitch, Headquarters Fifth Army, Chicago, IL:
>> copy of personal letter dated January 12, 1950,
>> provided by C. Scott, May 13, 2005

> I am sure it [the proposed legislation] is something we have all
> hoped would never really come up…. I personally do not believe
> we are ready to accept male nurses in to the Army Nurse Corps
> and hope it will not come before this Congress.
>
> LTC Katharine Jolliffe, Headquarters Third Army, Atlanta, GA;
> copy of letter dated January 9, 1950,
> provided by C. Scott, May 13, 2005

However, medical officers, other military brass, and the ANA disagreed
with these opinions. Debate continued for several more years, but it was
Frances Payne Bolton (R-OH) who persisted more than any other politi-
cian. She introduced five separate bills to strike down the ban. Rep. Bolton
introduced HR 2559 (The Bolton Act), which the Congress finally passed.
President Eisenhower signed the bill in 1955 (Craig, 1956). That same year,
Lieutenant Edward T. Lyon was commissioned as the first male nurse in
the Army Nurse Corps (U.S. Army Medical Department, 2009). During these
years and beyond, three remarkable male nurses fought for the right for men
to more fully contribute to nursing.

Role Model: Leroy Craig

Not much has been written about Leroy Craig's life, but he was one of
the most important male nurses of the 20th century. Craig graduated in
1912 from the McLean Hospital School of Nursing for Men, in Waverly,
Massachusetts (Obituaries of Leroy Craig, ca. 1976). This school was one
of the first nursing schools in the United States that educated male nurses,
primarily in psychiatry (Tranbarger, 2007a). Two years later, in 1914, the
medical director of the Pennsylvania Hospital for the Insane formed a nursing school for men and named Craig as its first director. Craig's appointment
was historic. He was the first male director of a nursing school in the United
States (Pittman, 2005).

Most of the schools for men at that time focused on teaching psychiatric
nursing and caring for men with genitourinary problems. However, Craig felt
that these schools limited opportunities for men. Shortly after taking lead of
the school, Craig included one full year of general nursing in the program.
Graduates from his school were well-rounded and could seek many types of
nursing jobs (Pittman, 2005). Craig stayed on as the school's director until his
retirement in 1956. The school was closed in 1965, after 551 men graduated
from it in its 51-year history. He died in 1976 (Obituaries of Leroy Craig, ca.
1976; University of Pennsylvania Hospital, 2010).

Craig was the most influential early leader in fighting for men's place
within the nursing profession. In 1940, he reported that there were only four
accredited nursing schools for men in the country. Several other schools
admitted both men and women (Craig, 1940). In order to attract more
men to consider nursing and enter school, he described the opportunities
nursing could offer men. He encouraged men to become private duty nurses,
who were hired by families to take care of loved ones. Private duty nursing was once the largest nursing specialty, but with the rapid expansion

of hospitals from the 1920s through the 1940s, the number of private duty nurses decreased. However, men who worked as private duty nurses often cared for patients with mental health or genitourinary problems. Since these patients could be challenging, private duty male nurses made much more money than female private duty nurses who generally did not care for these types of patients. Craig also encouraged men to pursue industrial (occupational health) nursing. These nurses worked in factories and industrial settings. They offered first aid to injured workers and ran programs to keep the workers healthy. Since factories could be dangerous places, Craig believed employers would be more likely to hire male nurses than female nurses. Craig also believed that more men were needed in hospital nursing. He noted that the lack of male nurses meant that many hospitalized men were cared for by orderlies and attendants, since female nurses were not usually allowed to give private personal care to male patients. Although many of these orderlies and attendants were dedicated and skilled men, they lacked the professional knowledge that would allow them to give high quality nursing care. In contrast, female patients were always cared for by registered nurses. Craig stated that this inequality was leading to a men's health crisis in hospitals (Craig, 1940).

Craig's most important contribution was his fight to achieve men's right to serve as nurses in the armed forces. Beginning in the late 1930s, the Alumni Association of the Pennsylvania Hospital School of Nursing appointed a committee to meet with medical and nursing groups to push for legislation to strike down the military's ban on male nurses (Craig, 1940). Eventually, this group helped form the Men's Nurses Section of the ANA, which made Craig its chairman. This group was instrumental in forcing the nation's largest nursing organization to examine issues important to men and to lobby Congress for the right for men to serve as nurses in the military (Men Nurses and the Armed Services, 1943). In the following years, Craig worked with Congressional representatives and senators, including Rep. Bolton, to draft bills that would allow male nurses to serve in the military. He met personally with Surgeon General George Armstrong and chief of the Army Nurse Corps, Ruby Bryant, to advocate his position (Craig, 1956). When the meeting did not lead to action, Craig contacted President Eisenhower to garner his support for Rep. Bolton's bill. Craig fostered collaboration among members of Congress and organizations such as the ANA and the American Psychiatric Association. In time, the number of voices supportive of men's rights grew. This encouraged the Defense Department to not fight the bill. Craig worked for over 15 years to strike down the military's ban. His ability to bring many voices to his cause and his patience with the process were instrumental in achieving this milestone for American male nurses (Obituaries of Leroy Craig, ca. 1976; University of Pennsylvania Hospital, 2010).

Unfortunately, Craig and his supporters were not immune to the negative social stereotypes of male nurses held by the public and by female nurses throughout much of the 20th century. The worst of these stereotypes was the belief that all male nurses were effeminate or homosexual. Some believed that schools that trained men and women together would produce effeminate male nurses. Even some male nursing students believed that it was better to separate male from female students. For example, one of Craig's students wrote the following:

> Note, please, the *right kind of men* [his emphasis]. Right there is the justification and success of the Pennsylvania School.... It tries to turn out *men* [his emphasis].... The man who nursed was often frowned upon because he was an imposter, not a nurse, but an attendant or orderly of limited training and, worse still, sometimes lacking in *manliness* [his emphasis]. (Crummer, 1924)

In a letter to the *American Journal of Nursing*, Craig recommended that only a small number of schools should accept male students. These schools would focus on leadership and professional development, so that male graduates would be offered education and administrative positions that would provide salaries attractive to men. Also, Craig believed that only the best students with good character should be allowed to enroll and graduate from these schools. Craig (1945) stated:

> The nursing profession needs to promote.... Careful screening of applicants before admission and early elimination of enrolled students who seem lacking in interest or aptitude. Particular emphasis should be placed on the importance of selecting men students who are definitely masculine. (p. 960)

Craig was quite worried about the damage that the negative stereotypes could have on male nurses. In the early years of the 20th century, male nurses had a reputation for being drunk and incompetent. Whether or not this reputation was justified, Craig believed that all the stereotypes, including the stereotype that male nurses were effeminate, would prevent men from getting high-paying private duty nursing positions in the homes of wealthy families (Pittman, 2005). Craig set out to promote a highly professional male nurse image that would dispel the myths about male nurses.

Craig carefully screened all applicants to his school. Tranbarger (2007a) noted a conversation he had with Luther Christman, who graduated from the Pennsylvania Hospital School of Nursing for Men in 1939. Christman reported that Craig and his faculty conducted two-day interviews with all applicants. The interviews explored each applicant's intelligence and personality. Part of the interview included a lunch, in which each applicant was observed for his social skills and table manners. Craig believed that men with poor manners would not be good representatives of the type of male nurse who would be successful with wealthy and respected families. If accepted to the school, applicants were often employed at the hospital for a number of months before classes started. This allowed faculty to monitor the students' behavior. Students were required to participate in sports and to bring sporting gear and clothing to school daily. Craig assumed that men who engaged in sports would not be perceived as homosexuals (Pittman, 2005; Tranbarger, 2007a). Also, Craig implemented a strict moral code. Students were expelled if they were suspected of homosexuality or if they misbehaved on dates they had with women. Christman noted that of the 30 men who started school with him, only eight men completed the program and graduated with him in 1939 (Pittman, 2005).

Lessons for today's nurse

You might wonder why I selected Leroy Craig as a role model. Clearly, his policies toward his students would be unethical and discriminatory by today's standards. Some would argue that his policies made the negative stereotypes about male nurses even worse. However, we have to consider the context of the times in order to truly understand the actions of any historical figure. During the early decades of the 20th century, the status of men in nursing was at an all-time low. Post-Victorian ideas about masculinity and what was appropriate behavior for men and women had taken a strong hold. Few men were encouraged or supported in pursuing careers in nursing. Even fewer men were allowed to enter nursing school. With few opportunities and little approval from others for male nurses, it is possible that some men with poor work ethic and behaviors were hired into low-paying positions. Although these men may have been few in number, there may have been enough of them to continue the negative stereotypes in the eyes of many. I believe that a system was in place similar to the system in English hospitals before Nightingale became a nurse, where low status, pay, and expectations attracted a poor quality employee. If allowed to continue, this system might have closed the door to men in nursing even tighter than it already was at that time.

Like Nightingale, Craig hoped to improve the quality of patient care by producing a more highly educated and professional male nurse. Although his methods were wrong by today's standards, his approach seemed to have worked at that time to prove the negative stereotypes about male nurses false. His graduates made a strong impression on others. Craig (1940) noted that Helen McClelland, director of nursing at the Pennsylvania Hospital in Philadelphia, was opposed to men working as nurses on general medical-surgical units at first. According to Craig, McClelland stated

> … It was only a short time before there was a realization on the part of all concerned that there was a decided improvement in the service given to the men patients when they were cared for by well-prepared men nurses. (p. 669)

This improved care was similar to the improved care noted by administrators in previous decades when patients were cared for by educated female nurses.

Craig was the first substantial advocate for men in nursing in modern times. His voice was unparalleled in a time of rapid change for nurses and for health care. He refused to accept the direction others were setting for the future of men in nursing. Craig knew that change would not come through rebellion, but instead, by producing high-quality male nurses who would prove the establishment wrong. He used the institutional structures of his day (the ANA and professional journals) as venues to state his arguments for change. Although his efforts were not immediately successful, Craig's persistence and well-planned approach changed the minds of powerful individuals who were then able to move his position forward to a successful conclusion.

Craig was imperfect, but Craig teaches us the lessons of fighting for institutional change and professionalism. In the United States and around the globe, too many people are not having their health care needs met. The health care debate seems never-ending as new financial and political policies and the advancement of science and technology continue to change the playing field. Strong advocates are needed to push through necessary changes. Nurses make ideal advocates since nursing's primary mission is to provide care and comfort to those in need. Craig teaches us to have the courage to raise our voices and to have the patience for change, even if that change is a steep uphill struggle. Also, Craig teaches us to show professionalism in all that we do, including our advocacy efforts. A loud and dramatic voice may get attention on today's talk radio and television broadcasts, but a professional voice supported by intelligence, evidence, and etiquette is what will ultimately change minds and change policy.

Role Model: Luther Christman

Perhaps no other male nurse of the 20th century has brought more visibility to men in nursing than Luther Christman (Houser & Player, 2004; Pittman, 2005; Sullivan, 2002). After experiencing much discrimination himself, Christman devoted his career to stubbornly fight for men's right to participate fully in the nursing profession. Christman had vision, proposing many reforms that were ahead of their time. His ideas often fell on deaf ears, only to be adopted later. His contributions were significant enough that the ANA recognized him as a "living legend" in 1995 and inducted him as the first male nurse in the ANA Hall of Fame (Pittman, 2005).

Christman was born in 1915 and experienced much hard work and difficulty as a child (Pittman, 2005). At the urging of a pastor, Christman enrolled in the Pennsylvania Hospital School of Nursing for Men so he could follow his high-school sweetheart, who was enrolled in the hospital's all-female nursing school. Christman's life-long fight against discrimination started early. He protested illogical and unfair treatment of male nursing students by the faculty at his nursing school. Christman (1988b) remembers:

> I submitted a request to the members of the faculty of the school
> for women asking to be assigned to a maternity rotation so that I
> could be prepared in a manner akin to that of most nurses in the
> country. I was denied because of my gender. I questioned that
> because all of the obstetricians were men. Even policemen and
> taxicab drivers were being trained to handle emergency deliver-
> ies. "That's different," they said. I tried to persuade them that a
> male nurse would be more helpful in emergency delivery than a
> policeman, but they were steadfast in their decision. They said
> that if I was ever seen anywhere near the delivery room, I would
> be dismissed [expelled] immediately. (p. 45)

With a few scrapes and bumps along the way, Christman did graduate in 1939. He immediately applied to earn his bachelor's degree, but was denied admission to Duquesne University because he was a man. Discouraged, he took a job outside of nursing because he could earn more money to support his new wife. Christman joined the U.S. Maritime Service when World War II broke out. Here he encountered his next struggle—the ban on men serving as nurses in the military.

Christman sent a letter to the Surgeon General requesting that he be stationed in a battle zone to work as a nurse, but he received a curt denial. Christman then sent a copy of the letter to every U.S. senator and appealed to local newspapers for support. Several newspapers ran articles in support of lifting the ban on men in the military nurse corps. The Pinella County (Florida) District Nurses Association endorsed Christman's position, but the Army Nurse Corps fought this endorsement. Christman (1988b) wrote later that

> A nurse from the Army Nurse Corps subsequently appeared at one of their [Pinella County District Nurses Association] meetings to chide them about that move. Her position was that if men were commissioned, all the senior women nurse officers would immediately be demoted and replaced by men. (p. 46)

Christman continued to be a strong advocate for lifting the ban until the ban was eventually struck down in 1955.

After the war, Christman again tried to earn his bachelor's degree. He returned to the University of Pennsylvania, but was told that if he enrolled, he would automatically fail every course because the university would never graduate a man from the nursing school. He applied to Temple University where he was granted admission and earned his bachelor's degree in 1947 (Christman, 1988b). With his bachelor's degree, Christman was able to pursue jobs in nursing leadership. Christman accepted an administrative position at Yankton State Hospital in South Dakota early in his career. While there, he was successful in obtaining better salaries for nurses and fought local discriminatory practices by offering jobs to Native Americans (Houser & Player, 2004; Pittman, 2005; Sullivan, 2002).

As the 1960s approached, Christman pursued higher education again. He earned his master's degree in clinical psychology and his doctoral degree in anthropology and sociology at Michigan State University. While attending graduate school, Christman was elected president of the Michigan Nurses Association. At the time, nurses' salaries were quite low, which prompted many nurses to leave nursing for higher-paying jobs. This resulted in a nursing shortage. As president, Christman negotiated, and even did some arm-twisting, with the Michigan Hospital Association to increase nurses' salaries by 10% in order to bring nurses back to nursing. The strategy worked. The number of nurses with active licenses in Michigan rose from 14,000 to 21,000 in two years (Christman, 1988b). After receiving his doctorate, Christman was offered the position of Dean of the School of Nursing at Vanderbilt University. When he accepted the position, Christman became the first male dean of a university school of nursing in the United States. Christman was the first dean to hire African American women teachers in Vanderbilt's history (Pittman, 2005). Five years later, Christman was asked to open the new school of nursing at Rush University in Chicago. While serving as dean at these two universities, Christman did much to advance nursing. Among his accomplishments, he

1. implemented and refined the faculty practice model for nursing. Under this model, faculty continue to work as expert clinicians, similar to the faculty model used in most schools of medicine.
2. implemented his Unification Model. This model included the faculty practice model, but also had graduate nursing students work side-by-side with medical students so that each may learn from each other. This approach is now recommended by groups such as the Institute of Medicine.
3. planted the seeds for the development of master nurse clinicians, including nurse practitioners, who would be educated at the graduate degree level.
4. developed the primary nurse model of care, in which individual registered nurses oversee all the nursing care given to a specific patient.
5. developed the Doctor of Nursing Science-Doctor of Philosophy degree to prepare future nurse scholars, researchers, and leaders.
6. started a community nursing service that gave patients a well-organized system of health care (Christman, 1988b; Houser & Player, 2004).

Many of Christman's ideas were revolutionary and not easily accepted by his female nurse leader colleagues. For example, in 1964, Christman proposed the formation of an academy of nursing. This academy was designed to encourage the advancement of nursing knowledge and health policy. The proposal was soundly defeated, but the academy formed nonetheless nine years later. Another example is found in Christman's proposal to develop a master's degree in psychiatry in order to prepare advanced nurse clinicians. This program was designed to use the Unification Model described above. He collaborated with Dr. Ewald Busse, a psychiatrist from Duke University. Dr. Busse was excited about the possibility of developing a nonphysician clinician who could provide much needed service to patients with mental health disorders. However, when the National League of Nursing (an organization that accredits nursing schools) heard of the proposal, they threatened to take back Duke University's accreditation unless it dropped the proposed program. It's not clear to me why the league objected to this proposal at the time, but I suspect some nurse leaders were fearful this program would prepare clinicians more like physicians and less like nurses. Christman appealed to the ANA, but received no support. Since nursing was not willing to work with physicians, the medical school developed a physician's assistant program instead. Nursing lost a golden opportunity for interdisciplinary collaboration. It wouldn't be until years later that nursing adopted graduate education for advanced nurse clinicians nationwide (Houser & Player, 2004).

Perhaps Christman's most important contribution was the creation of the American Assembly for Men in Nursing (AAMN). In 1971, Steve Miller, a nurse from Michigan, saw the need to form an organization for male nurses.

Christman was invited to join the group to help with its development. There was much interest in the group at the beginning, but the group floundered after a couple of years. In 1974, Christman reorganized the group as the American Male Nurses Association. The original purpose of the group was to fight discrimination and recruit more men into nursing. Christman believed that nursing would be strengthened as a profession by increasing the voice and visibility of men in nursing (Tranbarger, 2007b). As the organization grew, its focus broadened to include other goals, such as strengthening men's professional development as nurses and providing a forum for professional debate of issues. The group changed its name to AAMN in 1981. In 2004, AAMN became nursing's only formal voice and advocate to increase men's health research, policy, and education. Over the years, AAMN has issued a number of position statements and white papers on topics such as gender equality in nursing education, the use of gender-neutral language, combating negative images of nursing in the media, and the need to include men's health content in all nursing schools. In 2010, AAMN had 28 local and regional chapters nationwide. Christman retired in 1987 (Pittman, 2005). He continued to serve as the AAMN Chairman of the Board (AAMN, 2010a) until his death in 2011.

Lessons for today's nurse

Throughout his career, Christman fought like a warrior against discrimination. He fought his battles with determination, logical arguments, and sometimes, with a bit of humor. Not all his battles resulted in immediate victory. Many of his proposals were realized only with the passage of time. Other positions he took, such as a single standard for nursing education, continue to be a dream, much to the harm of the nursing profession. Some of his battles left Christman permanently scarred. He never got over his unsuccessful attempt to become the first male president of the ANA due to slanderous rumors and fear-mongering among the female members at the time (Pittman, 2005). It would be understandable if his challenges and defeats had turned Christman away from nursing in disgust, but they never did. Christman continued to fight, even in retirement, for men's rightful place in nursing and for ideas that would move the whole profession forward.

Christman teaches us to refuse to be knocked down when we try to move the profession forward. In his early years, Christman fought tirelessly for his right to be educated as a nurse to the highest possible level. He refused to accept that men had no place in nursing. Later, he refused to allow bigotry to prevent employment opportunities for minorities, refused to accept that nurses should only receive low levels of education, and refused to believe that nurses should serve beneath the physician instead of at the physician's side as an equal partner. The nursing elite through much of the 20th century saw Christman as a thorn in their sides—a real troublemaker. But Christman's power and eventual success did not come from troublemaking. Instead, his success came from the logic and clarity of thought that supported his positions. His critics could not fight his mind or his determination, and we are all the better for it.

Role Model: Joe Hogan

Not much has been written about Joe Hogan, and most nurses have never heard of him. Yet Hogan's refusal to accept the status quo did more to guarantee men's footing in the doors of American nursing schools than any other nurse before him. Hogan was a registered nurse working as a surgical supervisor in a medical center in Mississippi. He had an associate's degree in nursing, but he wanted to get his bachelor's degree so that he would be eligible for a promotion and graduate school. The only school offering an associate's-to-bachelor's nursing program in Hogan's area was Mississippi University for Women (MUW) in Columbus, MS, and MUW only admitted women. MUW believed that sex-segregated classrooms provided an ideal environment for women to learn (Greenlaw, 1982; Vance, 2008).

When Hogan applied to the nursing school in 1979, his application was rejected. MUW told Hogan that he could audit the courses if he wished, but he would not receive credit for the classes. This option would not give him the nursing degree he wanted. Hogan was told that he could go to other universities that allowed men to enroll. Two universities in Hattiesburg and Jackson offered similar nursing programs, but for Hogan to attend either of these universities, he would have to quit his job and move, or commute 294 or 356 miles round trip each day for class. Female nurses living in his area did not face this type of hardship (Greenlaw, 1982; Vance, 2008).

Hogan refused this offer and sued the State of Mississippi for violation of the equal protection clause of the Fourteenth Amendment of the U.S. Constitution. The District Court ruled against Hogan, stating that the state had a legitimate interest in providing educational opportunities with sex-segregated programs. Hogan appealed this decision and it was taken to the Court of Appeals for the Fifth Circuit. The Court of Appeals reversed the lower court's decision on June 5, 1981, and within two months, MUW was ordered to enroll any qualified student regardless of sex (Cornell University Law School, 2010; Greenlaw, 1982; Vance, 2008).

On August 25, 1981, Hogan, accompanied by his lawyer, came to the registration office and enrolled for classes. He was the first male to enroll in classes for credit in MUW's nearly 100-year history. However, by October 30, Hogan had withdrawn from his classes. He stated that he had not realized how difficult it would be to return to school while continuing to work full-time. The next semester, Hogan tried again. He completed the semester, but never returned to MUW to complete his degree (Vance, 2008).

During Hogan's last semester at MUW, the state appealed the court's decision. Before the appeal could be heard, the Supreme Court agreed to take up the case. The case went before the High Court on March 22, 1982. Much to the surprise of many, the Supreme Court struck down the ban on male enrollment at MUW on July 1, 1982 (Cornell University Law School, 2010; Greenlaw, 1982; Vance, 2008). In the hearing, the Supreme Court required the state to meet a two-step test to justify gender discrimination in light of the equal protection clause of the U.S. Constitution. The first step was for the state to show an important governmental objective for gender classification; and the second step was to show that discrimination was necessary to meet that objective. In a narrow 5–4 decision, the court ruled that the state failed to meet these tests. Although the court recognized the potential benefit of educational affirmative action, the state failed to show that females were disadvantaged in gaining admission to nursing school or in obtaining jobs as nurses. Ironically, it was Justice Sandra Day O'Connor, the first female U.S. Supreme Court justice, who wrote the majority opinion in this case (Greenlaw, 1982). In contrasting this case to previous cases in which violation of the equal protection clause was justified, O'Connor stated:

> In sharp contrast, Mississippi has made no showing that women lacked opportunities to obtain training in the field of nursing or to attain positions of leadership in that field when the MUW School of Nursing opened its door, or that women currently are deprived of such opportunities. In fact, in 1970, the year before the School of Nursing's first class enrolled, women earned 94% of the nursing baccalaureate degrees conferred in Mississippi and 98.6% of the degrees earned nationwide. That year was not an aberration; one decade earlier, women had earned all the nursing degrees conferred in Mississippi.... Rather than compensate for discriminatory barriers faced by women, MUW's policy of excluding males from admission to the School of Nursing tends to perpetuate the stereotyped view of nursing as an exclusively woman's job. By assuring that Mississippi allots more openings in its state-supported nursing schools to women than it does men, MUW's admissions policy lacks credibility to the old view that women, not men, should become nurses, and makes the assumption that nursing is a field for women a self-fulfilling prophecy.
> (Cornell University Law School, 2010, para. 21–22)

As a result of this decision, publically funded schools of nursing could no longer bar men from full admission in their programs. How the ruling applied to private nursing schools that received federal funds was unclear at the time (Greenlaw, 1982).

There is disagreement as to why Hogan only finished one semester (Vance, 2008). Newspapers in Mississippi reported that he was doing well in his coursework and was well treated by the MUW community. National papers reported a very different story. The *Philadelphia Inquirer* followed Hogan to some of his classes in April 1982. Reporter Julia Cass (1982) wrote that Hogan entered his morning class early and took a seat in the middle row. When the women came into the classroom, they left two rows on either side of him vacant. The paper printed a photograph of Hogan sitting by himself in the classroom. A few months later, when the Supreme Court handed down its decision, Hogan was quoted as saying, "It's finally over. I simply wanted to get an education" (Cantrell, 1982).

Hogan's actions forced MUW to open its doors to men and sparked a fierce debate between traditionalists and reformers (Vance, 2008). Reformers were generally people outside the MUW campus, who viewed the changes forced upon MUW as a triumph for equal rights. They also argued that allowing men to enroll would grow the size of the university and would have economic benefits for the city. (In the semester following the Supreme Court ruling, 132 men enrolled for classes [*Joe Hogan: The impact still spreading*, 1984].) Traditionalists were mostly students, faculty, and alumni who worried about a change in MUW's identity. They feared that allowing men to enroll would force the university to close. Although the emotions and rhetoric did not resort to threats of violence, most likely many people on campus shunned Hogan. He may have been shunned by people in town as well. It's easy to imagine the emotional toll on someone whose case is taken to the Supreme Court with such life-altering effects on a local community. By 1984, Hogan had left town and moved to Iowa (*Joe Hogan: The impact still spreading*, 1984). I have been unable to locate Hogan or determine if he is still working as a nurse.

Lessons for today's nurse

Hogan teaches us to display courage when we stand up for what is right. Although his voice of advocacy may not be as familiar to nurses as those of Craig and Christman, in some ways, Hogan's voice is more genuine. Craig's and Christman's most significant advocacy actions came when they were highly educated and in administrative positions of power. On the other hand, Hogan was a relatively unknown nurse working in a small Mississippi city. He simply wanted to advance his education and his nursing career. Hogan's fight truly represents a David-and-Goliath struggle. Hogan displayed great courage since his fight carried very great personal risk.

Hogan was not the first man to apply to MUW and be denied admission (Vance, 2008). However, he was the first man to fight back. He knew his denial was wrong and possibly illegal. His legal journey was emotionally draining. I'm not aware of any support he might have received from his coworkers or from the Mississippi Nurses Association, but I suspect Hogan felt very lonely in his fight for his rights. The challenges did not dissuade Hogan from his goal. He enrolled successfully in courses at MUW. Hogan's legal victory guaranteed that the slow movement of welcoming men into schools of nursing could not reverse course. Hogan teaches us that substantial change can come from an individual's courageous stand. His quiet start resulted in one of the most significant victories for men in modern nursing.

INTO THE FUTURE

In 2008, men made up 6.6% of all RNs in the United States (U.S. Department of Health and Human Services, 2010a). At the same time, more men were entering nursing school than ever before. Between 2001 and 2004, 9.1% of all students graduating from nursing school were men. That percentage rose to 9.8% from 2005 to 2008 (U.S. Department of Health and Human Services, 2010b). Men are now working in all kinds of settings. They are beginning careers that will yield many accomplishments. The stories of the male nurses of today and tomorrow are yet to be told. However, one man, Timothy Porter-O'Grady, is already blazing a path to greatness.

Role Model: Timothy Porter-O'Grady

Perhaps no other nurse has done more to prepare tomorrow's leaders to transform health care organizations than Porter-O'Grady. With incredible energy, Porter-O'Grady has accomplished much in his still-unfolding career. Porter-O'Grady earned his associate's degree in nursing in 1973 at Lower Columbia College in Longview, Washington. He immediately sought higher education, earning his bachelor's degree in nursing in 1975 from Seattle University, and his master's degree in nursing administration in 1977 from the University of Washington. While earning his master's degree, Porter-O'Grady worked as a nursing supervisor at Providence Medical Center in Seattle. Within three years, he assumed greater administrative responsibilities and became a national consultant on hospital administration. From 1980 to 1985, Porter-O'Grady led the development of a successful model for hospital leadership and shared governance (a model of shared power between employees and management) at St. Joseph's Hospital in Atlanta, Georgia. This model was instrumental in the hospital's recognition as a "magnet" hospital. (Magnet status is nursing's highest honor for a hospital. It is given to those hospitals with the highest quality of nursing care and working standards for nurses.)

Since 1985, Porter-O'Grady has served as a senior partner for his own consulting firm. He and his partners provide worldwide consultation services to health care organizations in human relations, mediation, operational management, and media services. He has earned doctoral degrees in education and in organizational leadership. He is board-certified as a nurse executive and a clinical nurse specialist in gerontology (the care of older adults). He also teaches at several universities (*Tim Porter-O'Grady*, 2010). Porter-O'Grady earned the AAMN's Luther Christman award in 2000. This award recognizes those who have made a substantial contribution to nursing and have made a significant positive reflection on men in nursing (American Assembly for Men in Nursing, 2010b).

Perhaps Porter-O'Grady's most important accomplishment is his writing. To date, he has authored more than 175 professional journal articles and 21 books (*Tim Porter-O'Grady*, 2010). Seven of these books have earned the *American Journal of Nursing* Book of the Year award, which recognizes books that make a substantial contribution to the nursing profession. Most of Porter-O'Grady's books focus on leadership and health care management. His books target nurses in all stages of their professional journeys, from a beginning nursing student to the seasoned nurse executive. One text, *Quantum Leadership: A Textbook of New Leadership* (2003, Jones and Bartlett) has become a "must have" for all health care leaders. More recent editions of this book were released in 2007 and 2011. In these books, he challenges nurses to embrace a new reality, in which step-by-step thinking is replaced by looking at the whole picture or system where the value of work is the outcome or end-product, not conformity to a process or tradition and where chaos is recognized as a means to force us to leave behind those things that get in the way of moving forward (Porter-O'Grady & Malloch, 2003). Porter-O'Grady has written much on *quantum leadership* in nursing.

Although there are multiple definitions for quantum leadership, McCauley (2005) described it as a style of discovery. Quantum leaders are always exploring and staying open to new possibilities. Porter-O'Grady and Malloch (2003) stated that today's nurse leaders "…must engage with [an] unfolding reality, perceive it, note its demands and implications, translate it for others, and then guide others into action…" (p. 7). Quantum leadership also recognizes that everything in health care is linked. What happens in one part of a health care organization influences what happens in another part of the organization. Dissatisfaction or inefficiencies in one department can make the work of another department difficult. Today's leaders, then, must be able to create ways that departments can share knowledge and resources and foster teamwork and cooperation.

More recently, Porter-O'Grady and Malloch (2009) noted that nurses must be leaders of innovation. In order to achieve the best outcomes, innovation leaders must adopt a new way of thinking and acting in order to mobilize the creativity and passions of health care workers. In health care, innovation leaders must develop skills that help empower workers to form innovation teams. These teams can explore best practices that result in high-quality care and health outcomes. Also, leaders must be skilled in building relationships both within and between teams from other health professions. These multiple teams must work as a community whose common goal is to provide the best and most comprehensive care to patients (Porter-O'Grady, Clark, & Wiggins, 2010).

Porter-O'Grady's work is not yet done. He continues to work tirelessly to encourage nurses to develop quantum leadership skills so that they may be key players in changing health care organizations into innovative, nimble, high-quality entities. It will be sometime in the future before we can determine the overall positive effect he has had on advancing the profession of nursing and improving the quality of health care.

Lessons for today's nurse

Porter-O'Grady provides two valuable lessons: the need to continue our education and the ability to think beyond the immediate work of individual nurses. First, Porter-O'Grady did not pause after earning his associate's degree. He continued to stay in school and quickly earn his master's degree. Clearly, Porter-O'Grady has talent, energy, and motivation, but without his higher levels of education, he would not have been able to assume such impressive levels of leadership within five years of earning his nursing license. Nurses have many reasons for not returning to school and returning to school is not always easy. Many nurses must juggle jobs, family, and school commitments at the same time. Porter-O'Grady was no exception. He worked as a staff nurse while earning his bachelor's degree and as a nursing supervisor while earning his master's degree. Despite the challenges, earning advanced degrees while we are still young enables us to push our careers quickly and advance farther than if we return to school later in our careers. It's not just increased knowledge that we gain from staying in school, but broader perspectives as well. In order to be good leaders, we have to be able to see the big picture, understand human behavior at a deeper level, be able to predict challenges before they land at your feet, and know how to find the answers to complicated problems. Higher levels of education afford us the opportunity to acquire these essential skills.

Second, Porter-O'Grady teaches us that transforming health care into a system that effectively improves the quality of people's lives requires well-functioning teams, not just great nurses. Many role models guide us on how to be the best nurses we can be. This is important, but it is not enough. The needs of patients are too complex to be fully addressed by just one profession. Nor can these needs be met by the teams of days gone by where the physician was captain and everyone else followed his orders. Today, physicians, nurses, therapists, social workers, pharmacists, information specialists, scientists, spiritual guides, life coaches, and untold numbers of technicians must work in concert with each other. Each member of today's team must be accountable to contribute much, and if need be, step in and lead the team in a new direction. Each member of today's team must feel powerful enough to speak up when something's not right or when something's missing. Each member of today's team must communicate, teach, and problem-solve in ways far more advanced than was required of health care workers a generation ago. Due to our closeness to patients and our long history of care, Porter-O'Grady believes that nurses are situated ideally to meet the demands asked of us by this new reality. Porter-O'Grady encourages us to think beyond ourselves and understand the systems that swirl around us. Porter-O'Grady challenges us to become the nurses of the future.

SUMMARY

Nursing's history is rich. It follows the history of humans, with all its twists and turns throughout the centuries. From the very beginning, women have sacrificed much and worked tirelessly to care for the sick and needy and create the nursing profession as we know it today. In books and films, and when we visit our health providers, we experience the amazing women we know as nurses. These women inspire us. They serve as role models to young people looking for meaningful careers.

Also, from the very beginning, men have sacrificed and worked tirelessly for nursing. However, men's contributions have gone mostly unnoticed. Often, authors have chosen to write about female nurses only. Few teachers and scholars tell the stories of male nurses to their students. This has caused some men to ask how they fit into nursing and even wonder if they belong in nursing at all. This chapter showcases eight impressive male nurses. Each of these men is a role model.

Role models help us through the struggles we face; and men face some unique struggles in nursing. Their stories and ideas help us problem-solve, guide us to a better place, and feel less alone in our struggles. Many authors report the benefit of role models, particularly for people who don't fit into the mainstream. For example, role models help troubled children, Black students, and women be more successful (Brown, 2006; Maylor, 2009; Quimby & DeSantis, 2006). In addition, many researchers believe that role models who share the same gender may have the best positive influence on people for career development (Karunanayake & Nauta, 2004). This belief is called the "similarity hypothesis." People who can identify with their role models have increased motivation to succeed.

People benefit more if they personally know the role models and they have frequent contact with their role models (Skidmore, Dede, & Moneta, 2009). Today, there are many male nurses who can serve as role models for young men just starting out in nursing. But many of these men are hidden. They are working quietly in their jobs, often away from most nursing students and new nurses. Therefore, historical figures may be the first role models available to young men at the beginning of their career journeys.

Historical role models are ideal in helping young men learn lessons that shape the values that they will need to become excellent nurses. (Table 2.1 summarizes the lessons we learn from historical role models.) These role models help young men understand that men have always served as nurses. Their stories inspire young men to accept the challenges of becoming a nurse. Once young men have entered school and have moved into a nursing job, they will find new role models who will help them understand how to apply

TABLE 2.1 Historical Male Nurses and the Lessons They Teach Us

NAME	DATES LIVED	LESSONS
St. Basil the Great	329–379	Advocate for those who are vulnerable. Fight for social justice.
Brother Gerard	?–1120	Values must be put into action for the service of others.
		Use social customs as vehicles to put values into action.
St. Camillus de Lellis	1550–1614	It's never too late to change your life for the good of others.
		Make vocation the foundation for your nursing.
Walt Whitman	1819–1892	Make the client the center of your care.
Leroy Craig	1887–1976	Advocate for institutional change that will improve men's opportunities in nursing and improve nursing care.
		Always maintain professionalism.
Luther Christman	1915–2011	Stay determined. Refuse to be knocked down when advocating for what is right. Use logic, clarity, and intelligence as your weapons when you advocate.
Joe Hogan	?	Have courage when you advocate.
		One voice, no matter how small, can accomplish much.
Timothy Porter-O'Grady		Continue to advance your education.
		Meaningful change only comes when you think beyond nursing. Adopt systems thinking.

values in their day-to-day work. These new role models will help young men become great nurses and, in turn, become role models for the generations of young men to follow.

REFERENCES

Alexian Brothers. (2005). *Early history of the Alexian Brothers*. Retrieved from http://www.alexianbrothers.org/english/history/timeline.html

American Assembly for Men in Nursing. (2010a). *About us*. Retrieved from http://www.aamn.org/aboutus.html

American Assembly for Men in Nursing. (2010b). *Luther Christman award*. Retrieved from http://www.aamn.org/awluther.html

Bainbridge, D. (2001). Disappointed in article on men in nursing. *Canadian Nurse, 97*(7), 7.

Barnham, K. (2002). *Florence Nightingale: The lady of the lamp*. Austin, TX: Raintree Steck-Vaughn.

Bartfay, W. J. (1996). A "masculinist" historical perspective of nursing. *Canadian Nurse, 92*(2), 17–18.

Bester, W. T. (2007). Army nursing: A personal biography. In C. E. O'Lynn & R. E. Tranbarger (Eds.), *Men in nursing: History, challenges, and opportunities* (pp. 83–98). New York: Springer.

Brown, W. K. (2006). The value of role models in inspiring resilience. *Reclaiming Children and Youth, 14*(4), 199–202.

Bullough, V. L. (1994). Men in nursing. *Journal of Professional Nursing, 10*(5), 267.

Campbell, T. (1908). St. Camillus de Lellis. *The Catholic Encyclopedia*. New York: Robert Appleton. Retrieved from http://www.newadvent.org/cathen/03217b.htm

Cantrell, W. (1982, July 1). Hogan: He never intended to be an antagonist to tradition. *The Commercial Dispatch* (Columbus, MS).

Cass, J. (1982, April 11). Male liberation Mississippi-style. *Philadelphia Inquirer*.

Christman, L. (1988a). Men in nursing. *Annual Review of Nursing Research, 6*, 193–205.

Christman, L. (1988b). Luther Christman. In T. M. Schoor & A. Zimmerman (Eds.), *Making choices, taking chances: Nurse leaders tell their stories* (pp. 43–52). St. Louis, MO: Mosby.

Cornell University Law School. (2010). *O'Connor, J. Opinion of the Court: Supreme Court of the United States. Mississippi University for Women v. Hogan: Certiorari to the United States Court of Appeals for the Fifth Circuit*. Retrieved from http://www.law.cornell.edu/supct/html/historics/USSC_CR_0458_0718_ZO.html

Craig, L. N. (1940). Opportunities for men nurses. *American Journal of Nursing, 40*(6), 666–670.

Craig, L. N. (1945). Need for men nurses. *American Journal of Nursing, 45*(11), 960.

Craig, L. N. (1956). Another goal achieved. *Nursing Outlook, 4*(3), 175–176.

Crummer, K. T. (1924). A school of nursing for men. *American Journal of Nursing, 24*(6), 457–459.

Donahue, M. R. (1996). *Nursing: The finest art: An illustrated history* (2nd ed.). St. Louis, MO: Mosby.

Dossey, B. M. (1999). *Florence Nightingale: Mystic, visionary, healer*. Springhouse, PA: Springhouse Corp.

Evans, J. (2004). Men nurses: A historical and feminist perspective. *Journal of Advanced Nursing, 47*(3), 321–328.

Goodier, A. (1959). *Saints for sinners*. Retrieved from http://ewtn.com/library/MARY/STCAML.htm

Greenlaw, J. (1982). Mississippi University for Women v. Hogan: The Supreme Court rules on female-only nursing school. *Law, Medicine, & Health Care, 10*(6), 267–269.

Houser, B. P., & Player, K. N. (2004). *Pivotal moments in nursing: Leaders who changed the path of a profession.* Indianapolis, IN: Sigma Theta Tau International.

Joe Hogan: The impact still spreading. (1984, February 2). *The Spectator*, p. 6.

Kalisch, P. A., & Kalisch, B. J. (1986). *The advance of American nursing* (2nd ed.). Boston: Little, Brown, & Company.

Kalish, P. A., & Kalisch, B. J. (2004). *American nursing: A history* (4th ed.). Philadelphia: Lippincott Williams & Wilkins.

Karunanayake, D., & Natua, N. M. (2004). The relationship between race and students' identified career role models and perceived role model influence. *The Career Development Quarterly, 52*, 225–234.

Kelly, N. R., Shoemaker, M., & Steele, T. (1996). The experience of being a male student nurse. *Journal of Nursing Education, 35*(4), 170–174.

Kummings, D. D. (2006). *A companion to Walt Whitman.* Malden, MA: Blackwell.

Lascaratos, J., Kalantzis, G., & Poulakou-Rebelakou, E. (2004). Nursing homes for the old ("Gerocomeia") in Byzantium (324–1453 AD). *Gerontology, 50*, 113–117.

Leininger, M. M. (1991). *Culture care diversity and universality: A theory in nursing.* New York: National League for Nursing Press.

Mackintosh, C. (1997). A historical study of men in nursing. *Journal of Advanced Nursing, 26*(2), 232–236.

Maylor, U. (2009). "They do not relate to Black people like us": Black teachers as role models for Black pupils. *Journal of Education Policy, 24*(1), 1–21.

McCauley, G. (2005). *Leadership in a quantum age.* Retrieved from http://www.partnersinrenewal.com/articles/Leadership.htm

McSorely, J. (1907). St. Basil the Great. In *The Catholic Encyclopedia.* New York: Robert Appleton Company. Retrieved from http://www.newadvent.org/cathen/02330b.htm

Mellish, J. M. (1990). *A basic history of nursing* (2nd ed.). Durban, South Africa: Butterworth's.

Men Nurses and the Armed Services. (1943). *American Journal of Nursing, 43*(12), 1066–1069.

Moeller, C. (1910). Order of St. Lazarus of Jerusalem. *The Catholic Encyclopedia.* New York: Robert Appleton Company. Retrieved from http://www.newadvent.org/cathen/09096b.htm

Monk, M. (1984). Saints for the sick. *Christ to the World, 29*, 270–276.

Nursing in a Democracy. (1940). *American Journal of Nursing, 40*(6), 671–672.

Nutting, M. A., & Dock, L. L. (1935). *A history of nursing.* New York: G. P. Putnam's Sons. [*Obituaries of Leroy Craig*]. (ca.1976). Pennsylvania Hospital Nursing Collection, 1876–1995 (MG 3.14, Box 7, FF 121). Archives of Pennsylvania Hospital Nursing Section, University of Pennsylvania, Philadelphia, PA.

O'Connell-Cahill, C. (1991). Saint Camillus de Lellis. *Salt, 11*, 31.

O'Lynn, C. E. (2004). Gender-based barriers for male students in nursing education programs: Prevalence and perceived importance. *Journal of Nursing Education, 43*(5), 229–236.

Order of St. Camillus Servants of the Sick. (2010). *Homepage.* Retrieved from http://www.camillians.org

Pittman, E. (2005). *Luther Christman: A maverick nurse: A nursing legend.* Victoria, BC: Trafford Publishing.

Porter-O'Grady, T., Clark, J. S., & Wiggins, M. S. (2010). The case for Clinical Nurse Leaders: Guiding nursing practice into the 21st century. *Nurse Leader, 8*(1), 37–41.

Porter-O'Grady, T., & Malloch, K. (2003). *Quantum leadership: A textbook of new leadership.* Sudbury, MA: Jones and Bartlett Publishers.

Porter-O'Grady, T., & Malloch, K. (2009). Leaders of innovation: Transforming postindustrial healthcare. *Journal of Nursing Administration, 39*(6), 245–248.

Quimby, J. L., & DeSantis, A. M. (2006). The influence of role models on women's career choices. *The Career Development Quarterly, 54*, 297–306.

Roper, R. (2008). *Now the drum of war: Walt Whitman and his brothers in the Civil War.* New York: Walter and Company.

Rose, J. (1947). Men nurses in military service. *American Journal of Nursing, 47*(3), 146.

Rudge, F. M. (1907). Orders of St. Anthony. *The Catholic Encyclopedia.* New York: Robert Appleton Company. Retrieved from http://www.newadvent.org/cathen/0155a.htm

Sabin, L. E. (1997). Unheralded nurses. Male care givers in the nineteenth-century South. *Nursing History Review, 5*, 131–148.

Sire, H. J. A. (1994). *The Knights of Malta.* New Haven, CT: Yale University Press.

Skidmore, M., Dede, Y. U., Moneta, G. B. (2009). Role models, approaches to studying, and self-efficacy in forensic and mainstream high school students: A pilot study. *Educational Psychology, 29*(3), 315–324.

Sullivan, E. (2002, Third Quarter). In a woman's world. *Reflections on Nursing Leadership*, 10–17.

Tim Porter-O'Grady. (2010). Retrieved from http://www.tpogassociates.com

Tranbarger, R. E. (2007a). American schools for nursing for men. In C. E. O'Lynn & R. E. Tranbarger (Eds.), *Men in nursing: History, challenges, and opportunities* (pp. 43–66). New York: Springer.

Tranbarger, R. E. (2007b). The American Assembly for Men in Nursing (AAMN): The first 30 years as reported in the *Interaction*. In C. E. O'Lynn & R. E. Tranbarger (Eds.), *Men in nursing: History challenges, and opportunities* (pp. 67–81). New York: Springer.

University of Pennsylvania Hospital. (2010). *History of Pennsylvania Hospital.* Retrieved from http://www.uphs.upenn.edu/paharc/collections/finding/iphgeneral.html

U.S. Army Medical Department. (2009). *Proud to serve: The evolution of male Army Nurse Corps officers.* Retrieved from http://history.amedd.army.mil/ANCWebsite/articles/malenurses.html

U.S. Department of Health and Human Services, Health Resources and Services Administration. (2010a). *The registered nurse population: Initial findings from the 2008 National Sample Survey of Registered Nurses.* Washington, DC: Author.

U.S. Department of Health and Human Services, Health Resources and Services Administration. (2010b). *The registered nurse population: Findings from the 2008 National Sample Survey of Registered Nurses.* Retrieved from http://bhpr.hrsa.gov/healthworkforce/rnsurvey2008.html

Vance, M. (2008). *Fighting the wave of change: Cultural transformation and coeducation at Mississippi University for Women 1884–1982* (Unpublished master's thesis). University of North Carolina Wilmington, Wilmington, NC.

Villeneuve, M. J. (1994). Recruiting and retaining men in nursing: A review of the literature. *Journal of Professional Nursing, 10*(4), 217–228.

White, K. (2002). Nursing as vocation. *Nursing Ethics, 9*(3), 279–290.

Yam, B. M. C. (2004). From vocation to professionalism: The quest for professionalization of nursing. *British Journal of Nursing, 13*(16), 978–982.

Zinn, H. (2003). *A people's history of the United States: 1492–present.* New York: HarperCollins.

THREE

Does Nursing Put Out the Welcome Mat to Men?

I got my first job as a nurse at a local Veterans Administration hospital in 1985. At that time, most of the nurses I worked with were retired Army nurses or nurses still on active duty or in the Reserves. I found this job much to my liking. There was much structure, many policies and procedures that answered any questions I had, and a very clear chain of command. As a new nurse, I thrived in this environment. My nurse mentors demanded much of me. They taught me with a firm, but supportive hand. At that time, there were a number of male nurses at the hospital, but I was the only male nurse on my unit. I don't remember feeling isolated as a man. Perhaps I saw many other male nurses in the cafeteria. Even though we didn't work together, at least I knew they were there if I ever needed to talk with them. My coworkers treated me fairly. I was included as a member of the team from the first day on the job. The fact that I was male seemed unimportant to my coworkers; hard work and competence took priority, not my gender.

Several years later, I left the Veterans Administration and took nursing positions in other hospitals. I saw a more traditional division of labor in these other hospitals, with most male nurses working in the emergency department or intensive care units. Few men worked on the general medical units like me. Also, I noticed other differences. Teamwork operated differently in these other hospitals. Instead of everyone working together to get the job done, I noticed multiple, smaller teams on each unit that sometimes worked against each other. For example, the day shift nurses were often at odds with the night shift nurses. The nurses were at odds with the physicians. The nurses were at odds with the therapists, kitchen workers, and other staff. Cliques of nurses did not work well with other cliques of nurses on the same unit. The chain of command was fuzzy at best. Often, a nurse with many years of experience exercised more power and influence over others than did the unit manager. At these other hospitals, I experienced isolation as a male nurse for the first time. I didn't think, communicate, or work the same way as many of the female nurses I worked with. Sometimes, my gender seemed to be my most defining characteristic. What I found most distressing was that some of the female nurses seemed to give me a cold shoulder. I wondered, "Why are they so mad at me? What did I do?"

As a man, I could not, nor did I want to be, included as one of the girls. I was ignored when coworkers discussed fashions and shopping. On the other hand, some female coworkers would ask my opinion, as a man, on relationship issues they were having with boyfriends or husbands. When I wouldn't give my opinion, they became angry. Some women told me that they enjoyed days I was on duty. They told me that when I was at work, there weren't as many fights among the women, as if I provided some kind of a buffer. Other women told me that I was successful at work only because I was a man, and that men always had advantage over women. Clearly, these women did not enjoy working with me. I had trouble understanding my place in nursing. At times, I felt that my female coworkers enjoyed working with me. At other times, I felt resentment from some of my coworkers. I wished my coworkers would stop seeing me as a male nurse, and instead, see me simply as a nurse.

Over the years, I talked with other male nurses about their cold-shoulder experiences from female nurses. Some men had more unwelcoming situations than my own; others told me that they had no problems at all. Most men, however, did recognize an antimale sentiment within nursing, even though it might be simmering just below the surface. Usually, men faced this antimale sentiment for the first time in nursing school. Sometimes it was mild or expressed by only one female teacher. Sometimes it was very strong. Some men said they received poor treatment only at school. Once they became nurses and started working, antimale sentiment disappeared. Most of the men I talked to have learned how to cope with antimale behavior from colleagues, but this took time and experience. Men felt unprepared for this sentiment. It was never talked about in school. I later researched this point. I found that 48.6% of male nurses stated that their nursing program did not prepare them well to work in settings that had mostly female coworkers (O'Lynn, 2004).

Today, I think antimale behavior from female coworkers is on the decline. Some of the decline is due to an increased emphasis on workplace diversity and effective teamwork. Some of this decline is due to general changes in our society, where men and women are more accepting of each other in the workplace. Yet, I still encounter men who tell me that their gender becomes a target for female coworkers. Where does this antimale sentiment come from? In this chapter, I will explore this question. I believe that understanding the sources of antimale sentiment within nursing will help men understand negative behavior better and help men respond to it positively if it occurs.

PATRIARCHY AS A SOURCE OF ANTIMALE SENTIMENT IN NURSING

There are many reasons why nurses behave the way they do. One nurse may be cranky due to lack of sleep, worries about finances, or trouble at home. Cranky behavior may have nothing to do with the fact that you are a man. Some of us assume the worst when we receive rude behavior. We feel attacked when others criticize us, or even when others simply give us a cold shoulder. We must be careful not to let the rudeness of one nurse color our beliefs about nurses in general. Also, we must be careful not to assume that a nurse is rude because he or she dislikes us as a person. Instead, the nurse may be upset only with something we said or did.

Yet when men talked to me about antimale sentiment, these men talked about common beliefs and behaviors that they saw in more than just a few female nurses. Behaviors were seen over and over again, not just on days when a certain nurse was in a bad mood.

When many people have common behaviors that come from beliefs and values they share, we say that these people are *socialized* into thinking and behaving that way. In other words, a peer group, or even a whole society, shapes the way we think. In turn, the way we think shapes our behaviors. A common way to think about this is culture. People from the same culture share common beliefs, values, and behaviors. Adults teach and role model these beliefs, values, and behaviors to children and foreigners so that they learn the ways of that culture.

The beliefs and values of the culture are seen everywhere; in media images, family structures, and the jobs people take. Beliefs and values are displayed so commonly that many people become unaware of their presence. Yet their hidden presence still sends powerful messages. For example, many Americans value youth and beauty. This value may not be stated openly, but it is visible in the people pictured in magazine ads, movies, and television. The frequency of these images reflects the strength of this value. Of course, as a culture or group changes over time, new beliefs might emerge. These new beliefs and new behaviors become part of a new or revised socialization message.

Nurses are a type of subculture—a small culture that lives inside a bigger or national culture. Nurses have some beliefs and behaviors in common. Nurses learn these from their teachers, role models, and peers. In turn, these nurses teach new nurses the beliefs and behaviors. This continues the socialization process. Some nurses' beliefs are greatly respected by the larger society, such as nurses' commitment to their patients. Some beliefs are not shared by all nurses, but by enough nurses over time that a socialization process is revealed. I believe that antimale sentiment in nursing has occurred in nursing's recent history due to socialization. As nursing has changed over recent years, the socialization for antimale sentiment has become less; but it has not disappeared completely.

You might wonder why nursing would include antimale sentiment as a socialization message in the first place. As a subculture, nursing is also influenced by the larger culture or society. The beliefs and values of the larger society influence the values and beliefs of nurses. I believe that antimale sentiment in nursing comes from the historical oppression of women in our larger society. The oppression of women at the hands of men is called *patriarchy* (although women can adopt the attitudes of patriarchy and oppress other women also). Under a system of patriarchy, men have more power than women, and men's concerns and needs are given more attention than those of women. In more recent times in our history, women and many men have stood up against the injustice of patriarchy. The protests against patriarchy often come from another movement loosely called *feminism*. There are many versions of feminism, but all versions criticize patriarchy (Tong, 1989). I won't provide a detailed explanation of patriarchy and feminism in this chapter; these are complex structures. However, it is important for men in nursing to understand *some* basic concepts of patriarchy and feminism in order to understand antimale sentiment in nursing.

Gender issues in nursing stem from a long history of patriarchy in Western societies (Kagan-Krieger, 1991; Miers, 2000). Johnson (2006) stated that patriarchy is not created just from the behaviors of individual sexist people. Instead, patriarchy is a system that can only exist with the support and acceptance of *many* people within a society. Johnson explained that patriarchy is a system of ideas, symbols, and ways of doing things that are male-centered, male-dominated, and male-privileged. Patriarchy gives advantage and higher value to men and to those things associated with men. Patriarchy favors characteristics associated with men (e.g., aggression, competitiveness, strength) over characteristics associated with women (e.g., collaboration, gentleness, vulnerability). Patriarchy leads to an imbalance of influence and power between the sexes, and ultimately, to the oppression of women.

Patriarchy influences all aspects of daily life, so much so that it is often unnoticed and considered normal. For example, think about the traditional family which represented the American norm for much of her history. In a patriarchal system, the man is the breadwinner for his family. His career is valued, so he receives a salary. He is expected to leave home for work. The woman is expected to stay home and care for the house and children. Her work carries less value. She is not paid for her work at home. The man, with social worth and money, has independence; the woman without economic freedom is dependent upon the man's salary for survival. Since the man is able to leave the home for work, he makes social connections, gains knowledge, and seizes opportunities that are not available equally to the woman. These give the man advantage over the woman. With advantage comes power within the family and, ultimately, in society.

Patriarchy's Influence on the Role of Nurses

Patriarchy has shaped the traditional roles men and women take in the labor market. Patriarchy shapes these roles by valuing what is considered masculine or feminine differently (Kleinman, 2004). Specifically, patriarchy places value and dominance on work considered masculine. Although traits considered masculine or feminine differ from culture to culture and change over time, traditional and stereotyped ideas about what is masculine are familiar to most people. Falk Rafael (1996) noted that masculine traits in Western cultures include independence, strength, and logic. Feminine traits include dependence, tenderness, nurturance, and altruism. Patriarchal societies assume that feminine traits are best suited for caring for others and taking care of the home. Therefore, women have been limited to work in the home in many societies throughout history. Patriarchy places low value on these domestic roles (Evans, 2004; Falk Rafael, 1996; Reversby, 1987; Stoller, 2002). Even as women entered the workforce, jobs that needed traditional feminine traits (e.g., childcare worker, nurse) carried low status and low pay (Evans, 2004; Kleinman, 2004; Reversby, 1987). Nursing tasks have been viewed as a natural extension of women's household and family work (Cummings, 1995; James, 1992; Kalisch & Kalisch, 2004; Miers, 2000; Reversby, 1987; Stoller, 2002). Therefore, nurses and the nursing profession have been devalued historically (Kalisch & Kalisch, 2004; Miers, 2000).

Modern nursing developed in Victorian times, when many people believed that the role of women was to serve the needs of men (Ashley, 1977; Reversby, 1987). Prior to the Civil War, most nursing care happened in the home. Patients were cared for, usually, by female family members. Few hospitals existed back then. Physicians visited their patients in their homes. Only the homeless, those who couldn't be cared for at home, or the mentally ill went to the hospital. As medical science advanced, new treatments were introduced that greatly improved patient care. These treatments required hospitalization because they were too complex or dangerous to be given at home. Soon, nursing care began to shift from the home setting to the hospital setting. Women began to take jobs in these new hospitals. Other women also began working as private-duty nurses, working in strangers' homes to care for those who were sick. Unfortunately, society still believed that it was the *duty* of women to care for others, and that caring involved having a love for others and a love for service. These beliefs fostered a system that paid women very low wages for nursing work. In other words, people believed that women should serve as nurses out of duty and love, not for money. Since women earned low wages, nurses held much less status and power than well-paid male physicians.

Patriarchy's Influence on Nursing Knowledge and Behavior

In far earlier times, the lines between healers and caregivers were fuzzy at best. Both men and women held multiple and overlapping roles in health care. Starting in the 10th century, the University of Salerno in Italy began training physicians (University of Salerno, 2011). Over the next few centuries, other universities opened in Europe to provide medical education. Formal university education was an important first step in establishing medicine as a profession distinct from all other healing occupations. These first medical schools provided education in the arts as well as in the newly developing sciences. Students were able to share, critique, debate, and test new ideas with their teachers at these new schools. This allowed medical knowledge to grow and deepen. Soon, books allowed students and teachers to share medical knowledge even further.

Unfortunately, these schools did not allow women. Without an education and an academic environment, women were at a disadvantage in sharing their knowledge with others. Instead, women had to share their knowledge the old-fashioned way—by word of mouth or demonstration to one person at a time. Without groups of students and teachers at universities, and without access to books and printing, women's knowledge became invisible in the recorded histories of Western culture (Ginzberg, 1999). As men gained knowledge, they gained power, and they soon devalued the knowledge held by women. Sometimes, women's knowledge was even demonized as witchcraft. Eventually, medicine and male physicians gained power and control over health care (Kleinman, 2004).

As Europe emerged from the Middle Ages into more modern times, educated men proposed new ideas about the nature of science and how to gain and use knowledge. Eventually, these ideas became the foundation principles for the way many people view science today. Science is difficult to define because it comes in a number of forms (Polifroni & Welch, 1999). However, on its most basic terms, I believe science is a collection of theories, laws, facts, and data (information) that define, explain, and/or predict truth, reality, and how the world works. Science has purpose, whether it is used to gain more knowledge or is used to solve a problem. Educated men began to question and devalue old-fashioned knowledge that came from experience, tradition, or religion. They proposed that knowledge which came from logic and experimentation, then verified by testing, was the best kind of knowledge to understand truth and solve problems (Polifroni & Welch, 1999). This type of knowledge was objective, and was assumed to be true in all situations. Men held up this type of knowledge as *science*.

Since men defined science in their own way, patriarchy helped their type of science to flourish and dominate Western thought even into modern times. Feminist authors have named this type of science as *androcentric* (*andro-*, meaning man or male), since it highlights the interests and thinking of men. *Gynocentric* (woman-centered) science is knowledge that fosters creativity and subjectivity. Gynocentric science is created by interacting and blending your ideas with those of others. Patriarchal systems have claimed that gynocentric science is not credible, and therefore, not as good as androcentric science. Some have claimed that gynocentric science in not even a science at all, but rather, a form of art (DeMarco, Campbell, & Wuest, 1993; Ginzberg, 1999; Perry, 1994; Welch, 1999).

Emphasis on androcentric science influenced the education of modern nurses greatly. Most nurses in the 1800s were uneducated. Nurses were expected to carry out various housekeeping and assistive tasks (Miers, 2000). But with the introduction of new scientific treatments, hospital nurses required some training to carry out these new treatments. Exactly how to train nurses and what nurses should learn sparked much debate in the late 1800s and early 1900s. Some believed that nurses only needed to be shown how to perform treatments. Others believed that nurses needed at least some education in the sciences to better understand how the treatments worked. At the same time, nurses began to set their own course for controlling their education, although it would be some years before they had full control. Beginning with Nightingale, nursing embraced androcentric science as a way to improve a nurse's ability to care for patients. Acceptance of androcentric science was also a way to elevate the status of nursing in a patriarchal health care system (Gortner & Schulz, 1988; Holliday & Parker, 1997; Perry, 1994). Nurses began to learn anatomy, physiology, pharmacology, and other science fields.

Immediately, many male physicians loudly objected to the idea of an educated nurse (Ashley, 1977; Kalisch & Kalisch, 2004). Physicians feared that nurses could become as knowledgeable as they were in health matters. They believed that educated nurses could challenge their authority and power in hospitals. Since many of them believed that nursing was an extension of a woman's role in the home, challenging the authority of male physicians would be similar to challenging male authority in the home. Objections continued for several decades, particularly as more science was introduced into nursing classrooms. Ashley described many articles written by physicians in the early 20th century as highly critical of nursing education. These physicians believed that much of the education was useless, too difficult for the inferior intellect of women, and too similar to what men were being taught in medical school. Ashley quoted physicians such as William Alexander Dorland and Edward Ill, who stated that nurses should never be overeducated, that nurses must respect the superior intellect of the physician, and that nurses are never made, but instead, are born with the attitudes and natural instincts of a good woman. They believed that natural feminine qualities made a good nurse, not their education. In 1906, Dorland wrote an article in the *Journal of the American Medical Association* that encouraged his colleagues to restrict the education and duties of the nurse. He stated that nurses with too much knowledge were dangerous to patients, and that only physicians could judge what nurses needed to know (Ashley, 1977).

Despite physician objections, many schools of nursing opened, and these schools followed Nightingale's lead to teach science to nursing students. By the 1920s, there were nearly 2,000 schools training nurses in the United States (Reversby, 1987). However, physicians and hospitals still limited the amount of education nurses would receive. Most schools were housed in a patriarchal hospital environment (Cummings, 1995) under the financial control of male hospital administrators and boards. Hospitals held great power over these nursing schools since the hospitals controlled the purse strings. Often, physicians provided lectures to the nursing students, especially lectures on science. This gave the physicians some control over how much science would be included in the nursing classroom. Also, hospitals required students to work long hours in exchange for their tuition and room and board. (Many hospitals required students to live in dormitories at the hospital.) The long working hours left little time in the classroom or for studying (Reversby, 1987).

In addition to education, patriarchal structures shaped the behaviors of nurses. Physicians, hospital directors, and nursing supervisors created strict learning and working environments for students. The slightest infraction could mean dismissal from the school. Fear motivated students to follow the rules forced upon them. These rules required that students obey all superiors, especially the physicians. Since physicians decided what nurses could and could not do in hospitals, nurses were forced into a dependent role. Unfortunately, female nurses who were in charge of the other nurses created a cruel pecking order among students and gave preference to nurses based on favoritism and social class. This pecking order reinforced a value on obedience to superiors, whether those superiors were male or female. The pressures of subordination were too much for many students, forcing them to leave school or be dismissed in disgrace (Reversby, 1987).

In the early days of hospitals and nursing schools, female nursing students and female nurses became the surrogate wives, mothers, and daughters for the patriarchal hospital family (Ashley, 1977). Many hospitals required that nurses perform all housekeeping duties and do everything in their power to improve the comfort and ease of the physician's work. Nurses took on a maidservant role to the physicians, a role that became a stereotype for nursing that has still been difficult to shake off. Head nurses made sure her students and employees always knew that the physician was in charge. Kalisch and Kalisch (2004, p. 133) reprinted a poem that was published in 1896 titled *When Doctor's on the Floor*. The first stanza of this poem reads as follows:

Nurses moving quietly,
Voices hushed in awe,
All things silent waiting,
Obedient to the law
That we have heard so often,
But I'll repeat once more
"All things must be in order
when Doctor's on the floor."

The expectation for obedience and dependence continued for many decades. Even as a nursing student and nurse in the early 1980s, I was required to give up my chair at the nurse's station and offer it to a physician when he entered.

Few men worked as nurses, since very few nursing schools allowed men to enroll (see Chapter 2). In the early decades of the 20th century, the few men who went to nursing school were educated to care for patients with psychiatric illness or men with genitourinary problems. Often, men enrolled in male-only schools. Regardless, obedience to authority figures was still required of these male nurses. Their gender did not allow them equal footing with male physicians or other men in powerful positions. Nursing was the work of women; it did not matter the sex of the nurse. Minor infractions to the rules resulted in serious punishment for men as they did for women (Christman, 1988).

Schools closely monitored the moral behavior of students as well. Reversby (1987) reported that many students were dismissed for dating, flirting, or even speaking with men in a familiar manner. Nursing textbooks in the early half of the 20th century frequently listed desirable virtues for nurses. For example, Harmer (1925) stated that nurses are defined by their love and service to those in need. Nurses must be sympathetic, kind, cheerful, reliable, trustworthy, obedient, and willing to be guided by their teachers. Some 20 years later, Day (1947) repeated these virtues, stating that nurses must be women of unquestioned moral integrity and possess a strong spiritual motivation. Although rules governing moral behavior loosened somewhat in the 20th century, other behavior guidelines for students continue to this day. Most of today's rules require students display professional behaviors at all times.

During the early decades of the 20th century, many believed that nursing school should provide young female students a safe home-like environment in which students could develop a strong moral character (Reversby, 1987).

With this idea, nurse leaders began to create an image of nursing as one of ministry. Advertisements at the time encouraged young women to choose a devotion to helping humanity by becoming nurses instead of chasing the more attractive incomes offered to secretaries and clerks in the business sector. Nursing adopted the belief that women would be more fulfilled by accepting the traditional feminine role of caring for others. Reversby claimed that glamorizing a woman's duty to care for others in a religious-like fervor sealed nursing's fate in dependency and oppression. As America entered World Wars I and II, advertisements for nursing continued to emphasize women's duty to care, although the message changed from ministry to patriotism. In other words, advertisements suggested that women could fulfill their patriotic duty by fulfilling their duty to care for the sick and injured as nurses (Reversby, 1987).

For students who finished school in the early decades of the 20th century, finding a job that would pay a decent wage was very difficult, since new students were available to provide free labor in the hospitals. Some graduate nurses became self-employed, hiring themselves out to families for private duty nursing, but hospitals insisted that students were just as qualified as graduates for private-duty nursing. Hospitals hired out students to families at a cheaper rate than nurses. This made finding enough work for nurses even more difficult (Ashley, 1977). To make matters worse, physicians complained that the salaries of private duty nurses were too high and made efforts to lower nurses' wages even further (Kalisch & Kalisch, 2004). Physicians and hospitals opened up special schools to provide women minimal training for home care and private duty services. Since there were very few regulations at that time, women who went to these self-study programs called themselves nurses and competed with educated nurses for jobs. Without economic power, nurses had little power to change the system.

The trouble with finding jobs and the concern over the poor quality of nursing care provided by uneducated nurses provided the push for registration laws and nurse practice acts (Kalisch & Kalisch, 2004). These laws set education and nursing practice standards, which must be met in order to carry the title of registered nurse (RN). These laws were passed state by state over a number of years. Nevertheless, physicians controlled both the education and employment settings for nurses for the first half of the 20th century. It wasn't until the late 1950s that nurses, by in large, took full control of the education of nurses (Cummings, 1995).

FEMINISM AS A RESPONSE TO PATRIARCHY

Feminism is difficult to define since there are so many variations of feminist thought and beliefs (Evans, 1995; Miers, 2000). At its core, feminism criticizes patriarchy as a system that oppresses women (Tong, 1989). It strives to encourage society to value the unique characteristics and ideas of women equally to the value we give to men's characteristics and ideas. Here lies the potential conflict, what Evans calls the equality-difference debate. Although simplistic,

I might explain the debate this way: If women are to be treated equally with men and enjoy the privileges men experience, then must women become more like men in their ideas and behaviors? If women become more like men, then won't they adopt the negative aspects of patriarchy and negative behaviors of men? Yet, feminists propose that women have different, positive, and possibly superior ideas to social and political issues. So, if we make everything equal, how can we honor and value differences? How can we value diversity?

Evans (1995) stated that most feminists have moved past this debate because there may not be easy answers to the questions raised. On the other hand, Miers (2000) said that this debate has led to differences in opinions among feminists. Different opinions have created different groups of feminists that don't always agree or work well with one another. For example, liberal feminists are most concerned about issues of equality. They identify how men and women are treated differently. They fight to have all restrictions removed from women so that they may experience all available opportunities equally as men. Radical feminists place more emphasis on the differences between men and women than do other types of feminists. They believe that women offer positive and superior approaches to life. Radical feminists suggest that relationships between men and women are based in power and oppression. True freedom for women, therefore, may only be possible by separating women from men and male-dominated institutions that refuse to change. Other types of feminism recognize that gender is not the only factor for the oppression of women. Class, educational level, race, and culture comingle with gender in creating levels of discrimination for different types of women. Sometimes, these other factors create more problems for women than does gender (Miers, 2000). These different questions and ideas about feminism have led to complex and fascinating efforts to reduce the oppression of women caused by patriarchy.

Nursing's Response to Feminism

In modern times, there have been three waves of feminism (Evans, 1995). The first wave occurred during the late 1800s and early 1900s. The fight to obtain voting rights for women is the most familiar accomplishment of the first wave of feminism. Sullivan (2002) stated that nursing ignored first wave feminism for the most part. However, Holliday and Parker (1997) suggested that Nightingale was an important nurse feminist during the time of first wave feminism, since Nightingale's work was driven by her desire to escape the Victorian barriers that were imposed onto her, and not necessarily by a desire to care for others. Furthermore, Nightingale used her celebrity status actively to manipulate men in power to accept her reforms to nursing. Over the years, Nightingale grew impatient with the lack of education, political savvy, and inefficient organization of the feminists of her time. Her impatience led to her decision not to work actively with suffragettes to obtain voting rights for women (Holliday & Parker).

The second wave of feminism developed in the 1960s and 1970s and continued into the 1990s (Evans, 1995). During this wave, feminists challenged the limits society placed on women's roles more forcefully than they had in previous years. Activists succeeded in getting politicians to address discrimination to women in education, employment, social and family issues, and health care (Cummings, 1995). As opportunities for women opened up, feminists encouraged young and bright women to go to college and pursue careers in high-status and male-dominated professions, such as medicine and law. Feminists did not encourage women to pursue nursing careers, which they often viewed as a throwback to patriarchal oppression (Sullivan, 2002). This created some tension between nurse leaders and the growing feminist movement. According to Sullivan, many nurse leaders felt that if feminism was encouraging the most talented women to steer away from nursing, "… then we [nursing] should concentrate on recruitment and leave the political rhetoric to the radicals" (p. 184). Also, unlike many nursing leaders, feminists encouraged women to increase the amount and depth of their education. Nursing did not move to require students to earn a four-year bachelor's degree, unlike other professions dominated by women (such as primary education and social work). I believe that nurse leaders clung to a patriarchal system that allowed a lower level of education for its workforce, in part, because nurse leaders felt that women had some influence and power in the community college setting. In other words, if nursing education moved to the university setting (which was more patriarchal in structure), nursing would lose power in the education of large numbers of women. I agree with Sullivan that these responses to feminism from nursing have damaged the profession.

Other responses to second wave feminism have been more positive. During this time, nursing wrestled itself away from a role that was dependent to patriarchal medicine to a role that is more autonomous, distinct, and mature. Beforehand, nursing had already accepted androcentric science as a way to expand, clarify, and define the unique knowledge of nurses in a language that patriarchal institutions could understand. It was believed that acceptance of androcentric science would help nursing establish a scientific base that would be respected by others (Gortner & Schulz, 1988; Holliday & Parker, 1997; Perry, 1994). By the 1960s, nurse leaders claimed that nursing was a scientific profession (Chinn & Kramer, 2008). However, during second wave feminism, nurse scholars challenged the profession's eagerness to adopt androcentric science, since this type of science does not address the values and concerns of nurses and women as well as it should (Campbell & Bunting, 1991; DeMarco, Campbell & Wuest, 1993, Ginzberg, 1999; McCormick & Bunting, 2002; Perry, 1994).

As a result, nurse scholars gave more emphasis to the development of gynocentric science. In 1978, Barbara Carper published a bold article that challenged the overreliance on scientific knowledge (what she called *empirics*) for nurses. Carper suggested that other types of knowledge (such as artistic, ethical, and personal knowledge) have always been part of nursing, but had not received equal recognition and value (Carper, 1978). Since then, other nurse scholars have expanded on Carper's work. They have explored how to obtain and apply these other types of knowledge. Most important, these scholars claim that *all* types of knowledge have equal value and importance in nursing. Also during this time of second wave feminism, nursing developed a unique language to label their diagnoses, goals, and actions (Carpenito-Moyet, 2008). Advanced education programs expanded greatly. More and more nurses with advanced degrees began to enter the workforce and forge new roles and leadership for nurses. Advances in the knowledge base for nursing brought the uniqueness and the value of nursing to light as distinct from the male-dominated science and health care industry.

Third wave feminism began to surface in the early 1990s, primarily by feminists of color who criticized the limited viewpoints of Caucasian leaders of second wave feminism (Heywood & Drake, 1997). *Third wave feminism* is a controversial term since it implies that there is an end to the second wave and a beginning to a brand new direction by feminists. Some believe that the second wave is continuing to mature and develop, but others note that feminists now have new thoughts about the consequences of second wave feminism. These consequences include the backlash against some feminist proposals, criticisms that many second wave feminists have ignored other types of oppression (e.g., class, race, sexual orientation), and different agendas between feminist activists and feminist scholars. In addition, there are unanswered questions about the role of men who support feminism (Messner, 2000). Most feminists agree that feminism has matured into a movement that embraces great diversity in thought and priorities. Embracing diversity is not easy. Organizing people with different opinions and experiences to work together on common goals is challenging. How third wave feminism might influence nursing is still unknown, but the first two waves of feminism have influenced men's experiences in nursing significantly.

Feminism as a Source of Discrimination to Men in Nursing

Once a society has determined which characteristics are masculine, patriarchy attaches high value to those characteristics. Because those characteristics have value, patriarchy makes it very difficult to change ideas about masculinity into something different. In other words, it's difficult to modernize our ideas about masculinity (Levant, 1995; Messner, 2000). At the same time, things that are considered feminine are not valued as highly in a patriarchal system, and therefore, are easier to leave behind. This helps explain why it has been more acceptable for women to leave the home and seek careers than it has been for men to give up careers to stay home and take care of children. Our history of patriarchy has created some rigid, old-fashioned ideas. One of those ideas is that women make better nurses because women are better at caring for others; therefore, nursing is not an appropriate career for men. This old-fashioned idea allowed nursing schools to forbid entry to male students and block male nurses from serving as nurses in the armed forces (see Chapter 2). Patriarchy's hold on society throughout history biased many nurse leaders against the possibility that men should be nurses. A general negative attitude against men in nursing persisted for the most of the 20th century, establishing a norm of the female nurse. Although patriarchy established the beliefs that were used to discourage men from nursing, I believe that second wave feminism and its influence on nursing helped negative attitudes about men in nursing to strengthen.

In the latter decades of the 20th century, nursing struggled to separate itself from the patriarchal dominance of medicine. Nursing lifted up women's ways of knowing and perspectives that were historically ignored by men. Nursing focused much attention to research on women's health and family issues. Authors suggested that the traditional college education stifled students. They concluded that a feminist approach to the classroom would enhance student learning and better prepare students for their roles as nurses (Chapman, 1997; Krieger, 1991; Webb, 2002). As a result, feminist ideas and theories began to dominate nursing schools.

During this time, some feminist nurse scholars with antimale sentiment changed their message from wondering if men had the ability to be caring nurses to a more paranoid message that if too many men became nurses, men would destroy the nursing profession. In other words, male nurses in large numbers would reverse the feminist advances within nursing and convert nursing into a patriarchal, male-dominated profession. For example, Ryan and Porter (1993) noted that men were more likely to publish articles in certain influential nursing journals than were women. Ryan and Porter feared that men would have too much influence over what nurses learn and what nurses think, similar to what male physicians had decades before. They believed this would oppress the voices of female nurses. Others stated that men get preferential treatment in nursing. Increasing the number of men in nursing will only worsen this reality. For example, men may use patriarchal structures in health care settings to position themselves unfairly for improved status or promotion (Evans, 1997; Inman, 1998; Williams, 1989). Male nurses take advantage of their relationships with female colleagues, teachers, and administrators to propel them into jobs that are more masculine, such as fast-paced emergency nursing or administration (Williams, 1989). Porter (1992) feared that nursing would become a gender-segregated profession in which men function as managers and leaders while women work in lower status bedside nursing positions. In the United Kingdom, Porter's fears may not be far off base. A recent study noted that men were overrepresented in management positions, though the percentage of men in leadership positions in acute care hospitals was still below 15% (Ford, Santry & Gainsbury, 2010). At the same time, hospital administrators denied discrimination against women. They stated that promotions were given to nurses with the best qualifications. Some of these administrators reported that women do not apply for the positions in the same numbers as do men. If fewer women apply, then more men will be promoted.

Worries over the negative influence of more male nurses foster an unwelcoming climate for men in nursing and encourages the continuation of discrimination against men. Much of this negativity toward men has been obvious in nursing schools (Anthony, 2004; Bell-Scriber, 2008; O'Lynn, 2004). (Chapter 5 details the barriers and discrimination men experience in nursing school.) However, negative feelings toward men are sometimes seen in the work setting as well. Simpkin (1998) named some of the behaviors of his female colleagues as "childish pettiness, sour grapes, professional jealousy, and downright bitchiness" (p. 32). Porter-O'Grady (1998, 2007) stated that men are often overlooked when nurses are selected for seats on committees or positions of leadership. Men continue to be turned away from employment opportunities in women's health, obstetrics, home care, and long-term care based on their gender (Coombes, 1998; Hawke, 1998). Hawke noted that some courts have found this discrimination to be legal, supposedly, to protect the dignity of female patients.

The different variations of feminism have shaped the beliefs and behaviors of female nurses differently. Also, a changing and more diverse society today interprets feminism in different ways. These differences help explain why some men experience little or no antimale sentiment in nursing, whereas others encounter much antimale sentiment. Some men have told me that many of the nurses they work with seem to hate men. Others have told me that only one or two nurses seem cold; the rest of the nurses they work with are wonderful. I believe we see this hot/cold presence of antimale sentiment on a national scale too. In recent years, there have been more calls to increase diversity in nursing by having more men enter the field (e.g., American Association of Colleges of Nursing, 1997). Yet today, no national effort to examine and resolve gender inequities in nursing has been launched. Sullivan (2000) stated, "We wait for men to apply for admission to nursing schools, and when they stay away, we figuratively shrug our shoulders at their lack of interest" (p. 253). I interpret nursing's continued silence on this issue to mean, at a minimum, that gender diversity is not a real priority for nursing. At worst, the silence suggests that nurse leaders still fear that men's greater presence in nursing will result in negative consequences for the profession, and possibly, for women.

The Response to Feminism by Men in Nursing

I suspect that most men in nursing are quite comfortable with the notion that women should have all the same opportunities as men. However, some men wonder if most women are comfortable with the notion that male nurses should have all the same opportunities as female nurses. Some men worry that if success comes to a male nurse, female coworkers will assume that his success was due to his male sex and had nothing to do with his skill and talent. This worry is not far off base. Evans (1997) and Williams (1995) published influential articles about the advantages male nurses have in a patriarchal health care system. These authors pointed out important points about how patriarchy hurts women. These authors did *not* state that discrimination against male nurses is acceptable; however, their articles fuel the fires of suspicion about male nurses who are successful in their careers. I believe suspicion can lead some people to adopt biased attitudes, which could lead to vengeful behaviors and discrimination if taken to the next level.

Other feminist themes put men in a more difficult spot. For example, themes that strongly emphasize how men have oppressed women can be difficult for some men to explore. Many men today may have some understanding of how women have been (and still are) oppressed by men, but these men may see themselves as very fair-minded. When these men experience very vocal and angry complaints about how men have mistreated women, they may feel like they are being punished for the sins of yesterday's men, or for the sins of some of the chauvinist men that live today. As Renee Heath states in Chapter 8 of this book, "…through no fault of your own other than being born male, you bear the brunt of your forefather's privileged position of power." For some men, this experience may make them retreat in confusion and anger. For other men, this experience may fuel backlash against feminism. Throwing accusations of oppression in the faces of male nurses clearly makes them feel unwelcome in nursing. These experiences may lead them to wonder about their place in nursing and how they might be able work with other nurses who are hostile to them simply because they are men.

Other men have responded to feminism by joining women in their fight against patriarchy (Messner, 2000). Yet, feminist men have a difficult struggle. Messner stated that men have to ask themselves, "With which [type of] feminism shall we ally ourselves?" (p. 61). Men who respond to feminism with backlash may consider feminist men as traitors or nonmasculine. On the other side, feminist men may face questions from some women who wonder whether or not they can be trusted allies because they are men. My experience has been that most male nurses avoid topics of patriarchy and feminism, regardless of how much they may or may not support feminist goals. Unfortunately, when antimale sentiment occurs in nursing, many male nurses remain silent. There may be personal reasons for the silence, but I believe many male nurses feel that they cannot protest antimale sentiment too loudly. They feel it is an argument they can't win with women, or that their protests will be interpreted as just another way men force their needs and beliefs onto women, thus continuing a patriarchal system.

ARE THINGS BETTER?

Despite negative attitudes toward men in nursing from both inside and outside the profession, the future for men in nursing may be brighter. More authors are writing about the barriers that men have faced in the profession and are publishing calls to reduce those barriers and recruit more men into the profession. Most of these authors offer suggestions on how to do this. For example, Oxtoby (2003) reported that more positive images of male nurses in the media are related to a steady rise of men entering nursing in the United Kingdom. In Texas, Williams (2002) reported that having male nurses meet with students at career fairs contributed to a sharp increase in the number of men entering nursing school. More studies that explore how to help make nursing more welcoming to men and how to encourage men to stay in the nursing field are greatly needed.

Recent studies suggested that more men and women today believe that nursing *is* an appropriate career choice for men (Bartfay, Bartfay, Clow & Wu, 2010; Buerhaus, Donelan, Norman & Dittus, 2005; Saritas, Karadag & Yildirim, 2009); however, these studies reported the opinions of nursing students. Nursing students may have more positive attitudes about men in nursing than do nurses from previous generations, but these students will become future nurses and bring their positive attitudes to the workplace. Of course, not all older nurses cling to old-fashioned ideas. McCrae (2003) noted that 73% of obstetric nurses had positive attitudes about men as labor and delivery nurses. McCrae believed that having past experience working with male nurses makes all the difference in accepting male nurses, even in a female-dominated setting like obstetrics. As more men work as nurses, gender may become less of an uncomfortable issue. In fact, McCrae noted that many of the patients she interviewed stated that they were more concerned about the nurse's experience and qualifications than whether the nurse was male or female.

Increased positive attitudes toward men in nursing and increased awareness of the opportunities available to men in nursing may be contributing to a greater interest among men for a nursing career. The percentage of men in nursing school is increasing, although still very slowly. In a recent survey, 11.4% of students enrolled in nursing baccalaureate programs were men (AACN, 2011). More important, more men are graduating from nursing school and entering the workforce. Between 2001 and 2004, 9.1% of all students graduating from nursing school were men. That percentage rose to 9.8% from 2005 to 2008 (U.S. Department of Health and Human Services, 2010). Another positive sign is the growth in size of the American Assembly for Men in Nursing (AAMN, 2001). AAMN is an organization whose mission includes increasing the number of men in nursing and fostering professional development of male nurses. At the start of 2011, AAMN had 28 chapters spread across the United States, a significant increase from the seven chapters that existed in 2001 (AAMN, 2001, 2011a). Over the years, AAMN has issued position statements and white papers calling for gender equality in nursing, the end to discrimination against male nursing students, the use of gender neutral language in nursing, the end of negative images of male nurses, and the inclusion of men's health content in nursing education (AAMN, 2011b; Tranbarger, 2007). Further information regarding this organization can be found on the AAMN website at www.aamn.org.

SUMMARY

No matter where you work, you are going to meet some coworkers who will give you a cold shoulder from time to time. There are many reasons why someone would do this to you. Often, those reasons have nothing to do with you personally. Your cranky coworker might just be going through a tough time. You and your other coworkers may simply be targets for this coworker's negativity. Giving this coworker the benefit of the doubt, having a talk with this coworker about his or her behavior, and offering this coworker some emotional support may go a long way in solving the problem, and in building teamwork. On the other hand, many male nurses report that there is an antimale sentiment floating throughout nursing. This sentiment is not universal; men don't experience this sentiment from all nurses or in all settings. Nevertheless, men state that they see and feel the negativity of antimale sentiment at some point in their nursing careers. Men report that they face this sentiment usually for the first time in nursing school. Antimale sentiment may follow men as they leave school and move into the workplace.

The commonness of antimale sentiment in nursing suggests that it develops from socialization. Nurses are socialized by society and by other nurses to adopt certain beliefs and values. These beliefs and values then lead to certain behaviors that are seen and experienced by others. I believe that a long history of patriarchy in our society has created a system of inequality that devalues women and things that are considered feminine. Patriarchy is responsible for the false ideas that nursing is not as valuable as other professions and that nursing is not an appropriate profession for men. Patriarchy creates a system of oppression. Some theories of oppression suggest that oppressed people sometimes participate in their own oppression (Cudd, 2006). Historically, some women in nursing have supported some patriarchal beliefs, and therefore, continue the oppression of nurses. For example, the use of power and fear to enforce a strict obedience to superiors, and the continuation of a belief that men shouldn't be nurses because nursing is better suited for women support certain patriarchal beliefs. The remnants of these beliefs generate some antimale sentiment from a few nurses today.

Feminism has grown stronger in fighting the injustice of patriarchy. Nursing has benefited greatly from the changes brought about by feminism. For example, nursing has embraced all forms of science in order to improve the knowledge and skill of nurses. However, feminism can lead to some antimale sentiment. Some forms of feminist beliefs may devalue men in order to lift women up. Although these beliefs may be in the minority, some men have accused feminism of sparking feelings of vengeance toward men. Today's men, in effect, must pay for the sins of their forefathers. In nursing, we rarely see open acts of discrimination against men stemming from vengeance. On the other hand, some nurses do devalue men as a way to lift women up. For example, men have been accused of trying to dominate nursing science when they publish articles, or have been accused of advancing their careers on the backs of women. Legalized discrimination against some male nurses still exists in certain employment settings. Male nurses see these realities as evidence of an undercurrent of antimale sentiment in nursing that still exists.

Many men are unaware of an antimale sentiment within nursing. In this chapter, I bring this antimale sentiment to light and explain why I believe it is present in nursing. My intent is not to deter men from pursuing careers in nursing. Instead, my intent is to raise awareness so men can be better prepared to confront antimale sentiment if they come face-to-face with it. If men are not prepared for the possibility of antimale sentiment, they may grow frustrated with their female colleagues and leave nursing school or their nursing careers. This will only strengthen men's minority status in nursing. Later chapters in this book will provide you strategies that you can use to improve all working relationships, including those with female nurse colleagues. Improved working relationships benefit everyone, including the patient.

REFERENCES

American Assembly for Men in Nursing. (2001). Chapters. *Interaction, 19*(1), 9.
American Assembly for Men in Nursing. (2011a). *Chapters.* Retrieved March 17, 2011 from http://www.aamn.org/chapters.shtml
American Assembly for Men in Nursing. (2011b). *What's new?* Retrieved March 17, 2011 from http://www.aamn.org

American Association of Colleges of Nursing. (1997). *Diversity and equality in opportunity*. Retrieved 2/11/2011 from http://www.aacn.nche.edu/Publications/positions/diverse.htm

American Association of Colleges of Nursing. (2011). *Despite economic challenges facing schools of nursing, new AACN data confirm sizable growth in doctoral nursing programs*. Retrieved March 17, 2011 from http://www.aacn.nche.edu/Media/NewsReleases/2011/enrollsurge.html

Anthony, A. S. (2004). Gender bias and discrimination in nursing education: Can we change it? *Nurse Educator, 29*(3), 121–125.

Ashley, J. (1977). *Hospitals, paternalism, and the role of the nurse*. New York: Teachers College Press.

Bartfay, W. J., Bartfay, E., Clow, K. A., & Wu, T. (2010). Attitudes and perceptions towards men in nursing education. *The Internet Journal of Allied Health Sciences and Practice, 8*(2). ISSN: 1540-580X

Bell-Scriber, M. J. (2008). Warming the nursing education climate for traditional-age learners who are male. *Nursing Education Perspectives, 29*(3), 143–150.

Buerhaus, P. I., Donelan, K., Norman, L., & Dittus, R. (2005). Nursing students' perceptions of a career in nursing and impact of a national campaign designed to attract people into the nursing profession. *Journal of Professional Nursing, 21*(2), 75–83.

Campbell, J. C., & Bunting, S. (1991). Voices and paradigms: Perspectives on critical and feminist theory in nursing. *Advances in Nursing Science, 13*(3), 1–15.

Carpenito-Moyet, L. J. (2008). *Nursing diagnosis: Application to clinical practice* (12th ed.). Philadelphia: Lippincott Williams & Wilkins.

Carper, B. A. (1978). Fundamental patterns of knowing in nursing. *Advances in Nursing Science, 1*(1), 13–24.

Chapman, E. (1997). Nurse education: A feminist approach. *Nurse Education Today, 17*, 209–214.

Christman, L. (1988). Men in nursing. In J. L. Fitzpatrick, R. L. Tasinton, & J.Q. Benoliel (Eds.), *Annual review of nursing research*. New York, NY: Springer Publishing.

Chinn, P. L., & Kramer, M. K. (2008). *Integrated theory and knowledge development in nursing* (7th ed.). St. Louis, MO: Mosby/ Elsevier.

Coombes, R. (1998). Jobs for the girls. *Nursing Times, 94*(9), 14–15.

Cudd, A. E. (2006). *Analyzing oppression*. New York: Oxford University Press.

Cummings, S. H. (1995). Attila the Hun versus Attila the hen: gender socialization of the American nurse. *Nursing Administration Quarterly, 19*(2), 19–29.

Day, M. A. C. (1947). *Basic science in the nursing arts*. St. Louis, MO: Mosby.

DeMarco, R., Campbell, J., & Wuest, J. (1993). Feminist critique: searching for meaning in research. *Advances in Nursing Science, 16*(2), 26–38.

Evans, J. (1995). *Feminist theory today: An introduction to second-wave feminism*. Thousand Oaks, CA: Sage.

Evans, J. (1997). Men in nursing: Issues of gender segregation and hidden advantage. *Journal of Advanced Nursing, 26*(2), 226–231.

Evans, J. (2004). Men nurses: a historical and feminist perspective. *Journal of Advanced Nursing, 47*(3), 321–328.

Falk Rafael, A. R. (1996). Power and caring: a dialectic in nursing. *Advances in Nursing Science, 19*(1), 3–17.

Ford, S., Santry, C., & Gainsbury, S. (2010, August 17). Top hospitals show bias for male nurse directors. *Nursing Times* [online]. Retrieved March 17, 2011 from www.nursingtimes.net

Ginzberg, R. (1999). Uncovering gynocentric science. In E. C. Polifroni and M. Welch (Eds.), *Perspectives on philosophy of science in nursing: an historical and contemporary anthology* (pp. 440–450). Philadelphia: Lippincott.

Gortner, S. R., & Schulz, P. R. (1988). Approaches to nursing science methods. *IMAGE: Journal of Nursing Scholarship, 20*(1), 22–24.

Harmer, B. (1925). *Textbook of the principles and practice of nursing.* New York: Macmillan.

Hawke, C. (1998). Nursing a fine line: Patient privacy and sex discrimination. *Nursing Management, 29*(10), 56–61.

Heywood, L., & Drake, J. (Eds.) (1997). *Third wave agenda: Being feminist, doing feminism.* Minneapolis, MN: University of Minnesota Press.

Holliday, M. E., & Parker, D. L. (1997). Florence Nightingale, feminism, and nursing. *Journal of Advanced Nursing, 26,* 483–488.

Inman, K. (1998). Male order nursing. *Nursing Times, 94*(32), 12–13.

James, N. (1992). Care = organisation + physical labour + emotional labour. *Sociology of Health & Illness, 14*(4), 398–509.

Johnson, A. G. (2006). Patriarchy, the system. An It, not a He, a Them, or an Us. In E. Disch (Ed.), *Reconstructing gender: a multicultural anthology* (4th ed., pp. 91–98). New York: McGraw-Hill.

Kagan-Krieger, S. (1991). Nursing and feminism. *The Canadian Nurse, 87*(8), 30–32.

Kalisch, P. A., & Kalisch, B. J. (2004). *American nursing: A history.* Philadelphia: Lippincott.

Kleinman, C. S. (2004). Understanding and capitalizing on men's advantage in nursing. *Journal of Nursing Administration, 34*(2), 78–82.

Krieger, S.K. (1991). Nursing-ed and feminism. *The Canadian Nurse, 87*(8), 30–32.

Levant, R. F. (1995). *Masculinity reconstructed: Changing the rule of manhood at work, in relationships, and in family life.* New York: Plume.

McCormick, K. M., & Bunting, S. M. (2002). Application of feminist theory in nursing research: the case of women and cardiovascular disease. *Health Care for Women International, 23,* 820–834.

McCrae, M. J. (2003). Men in obstetrical nursing: Perceptions of the role. *MCN, The American Journal of Maternal/Child Nursing, 28*(3), 167–173.

Messner, M. A. (2000). *Politics of masculinities: Men in movements.* Walnut Creek, CA: Altimira Press.

Miers, M. (2000). *Gender issues and nursing practice.* London, UK: Macmillan.

O'Lynn, C. E. (2004). Gender-based barriers for male students in nursing education programs: prevalence and perceived importance. *Journal of Nursing Education, 43*(5), 229–236.

Oxtoby, K. (2003). Men in nursing. *Nursing Times, 99*(32), 20–23.

Perry, P. A. (1994). Feminist empiricism as a method of inquiry in nursing. *Western Journal of Nursing Research, 16*(5), 480–493.

Polifroni, E. C., & Welch, M. (1999). Nursing and philosophy of science: connections and disconnections. In E. C. Polifroni and M. Welch (Eds.), *Perspectives on philosophy of science in nursing: an historical and contemporary anthology* (pp. 1–11). Philadelphia: Lippincott.

Porter, S. (1992). Women in a women's job: The gendered experience of nurses. *Sociology of Health and Illness, 14*(4), 510–527.

Porter-O'Grady, T. (1998). Nursing and the challenge of gender inequity. *Reflections on Nursing Leadership, 24*(2), 24–25.

Porter-O'Grady, T. (2007). Reverse discrimination in nursing leadership: Hitting the concrete ceiling. In C. E. O'Lynn & R. E. Tranbarger (Eds.) *Men in nursing: History, challenges, and opportunities* (pp. 143–151). New York, NY: Springer Publishing.

Reversby, S. M. (1987). *Ordered to care: The dilemma of American nursing, 1850–1945.* Cambridge, UK: Cambridge University Press.

Ryan, S., & Porter, S. (1993). Men in nursing: A cautionary critique. *Nursing Outlook, 41,* 262–267.

Saritas, S., Karadag, M., & Yildirim, D. (2009). School for health sciences university students' opinions about male nurses. *Journal of Professional Nursing, 25*(5), 279–284.

Simpkin, W. (1998). Gender-bashing. *Nursing Times, 94*(49), 32, 37.

Stoller, E. P. (2002). Theoretical perspectives on caregiving men. In B. J. Kramer & E. H. Thompson (Eds.) *Men as caregivers: theory, research, and service implications* (pp. 51–68). New York, NY: Springer Publishing.

Sullivan, E. J. (2000). Men in nursing: The importance of gender diversity. *Journal of Professional Nursing, 16*(5), 253–254.

Sullivan, E. J. (2002). Nursing and feminism: An uneasy alliance. *Journal of Professional Nursing, 18*(4), 183–184.

Tong, R. (1989). *Feminist thought: A comprehensive introduction.* Boulder, CO: Westview.

Tranbarger, R. E. (2007). The American Assembly for Men in Nursing (AAMN): The first 30 years as reported in Interaction. In C. E. O'Lynn & R. E. Tranbarger (Eds.) *Men in nursing: History, challenges, and opportunities* (pp. 67–82). New York, NY: Springer Publishing.

University of Salerno. (2011). In *Encylcopedia Britannica.* Retrieved from http://www.britannica.com/EBchecked/topic/519082/University-of-Salerno

U.S. Department of Health and Human Services, Health Resources and Services Administration. (2010). *The registered nurse population: Findings from the 2008 National Sample Survey of Registered Nurses.* Retrieved from http://bhpr.hrsa.gov/healthworkforce/rnsurvey2008.html

Webb, C. (2002). Feminism, nursing, and education. *Journal of Advanced Nursing, 39*(2), 111–113.

Welch, M. (1999). Science and gender. In E. C. Polifroni and M. Welch (Eds.) *Perspectives on philosophy of science in nursing: an historical and contemporary anthology* (pp. 440–450). Philadelphia, PA: Lippincott.

Williams, C. (1995). Hidden advantages for men in nursing. *Nursing Administration Quarterly, 19*(2), 63–70.

Williams, C. L. (1989). *Gender differences at work: Women and men in non-traditional occupations.* Berkeley, CA: University of California Press.

Williams, D. (2002). Looking for a few good men. *Minority Nurse, 9*(2), 22–27.

FOUR

Where Is the Starting Line? Getting Into Nursing School

Stacey Boatright

You're ready to move forward. You know your end goal is to start nursing school. You're finishing up the last course in your anatomy and physiology series, so you know the time is almost right for you to start nursing school. You have all the passion and motivation necessary to succeed, and you're convinced that nursing is your calling. The only problem is you don't know where to start. The stories you've heard about the competitiveness of admission to nursing school and the daunting application checklists you'll have to complete make it overwhelming. In this chapter, speaking as a dedicated student services professional who has worked solely in the realm of nursing school admission for my entire career, I offer an explanation of the realities of today's nursing school admission process. I will help you find the starting line.

From a young age, many of us have been asked, and asked ourselves, what we want to be when we grow up. The fact that you've done your vocational soul-searching and decided on becoming a nurse—that you've *finally* answered the question—must be quite a rewarding feeling! Now that your goal is set, it's time to get serious about the steps you're going to take to become a nurse, starting with how to get into nursing school. From my experience and research, I have one very important, though somewhat discouraging, message: Even though an individual may have a genuine desire to become a nurse, the reality is that not everyone will find the way to become a nurse. As I will explain in more detail, there are far more people who want to become a nurse than there are seats available in nursing schools.

Nursing school admission is an incredibly competitive arena. During the 2010–2011 academic year, there were approximately 255,671 complete applications submitted to entry-level bachelor's degree (BSN) programs across the United States, but only 101,060 applicants were accepted (American Association of Colleges of Nursing [AACN], 2012). This means that 154,611 applicants were turned away, or a 39.5% acceptance rate. Even further, AACN reported that 75,587 of the applicants who were turned away fully met the qualifications for admission. The point here is that having top grades alone is not enough to receive an acceptance letter. Likewise, making the application reviewers cry when they read your heart-wrenching story about why you want to be a nurse won't land you a seat in a nursing school on its own either. And, just because you're a Hispanic male and you know that every nursing school wants to admit an ethnically diverse class doesn't mean you're automatically on the acceptance list either.

Year after year, I see applicants who exceed every minimum numerical admission requirement (e.g., cumulative grade point average [GPA], science GPA, college entrance exam scores) but are denied admission due to a poorly written essay or troubling social skills during the admission interview. On the flip side, without fail, every year I see applicants, who appear to have the perfect personal characteristics, qualities, values, and motivations to become an exceptional registered nurse (RN), but don't meet the minimum grade requirements and are denied admission also. In today's nursing school admission world, if you want your application to be stamped and signed "Approved," then you need to prepare appropriately and make your application stand out from the rest. I have several tips and words of advice to help you get that approval letter.

NURSING IS H-O-T, HOT RIGHT NOW!

Quite simply, nursing is hot right now. Even though recent hard economic times have made it more difficult for some nurses to find jobs right after graduating from nursing school, many nurses are set to retire in the next few years. Combined with the growing health care market, there is a looming shortage of nurses that is well underway. This shortage offers nurses job security in contrast with many other professions. Nurses earn impressive wages and benefits. Also, once you're a nurse, there are many opportunities for changes, further education, and career advancement. There is no excuse for reaching a career plateau or rut in today's nursing. With all of these positives on the list, it's no wonder why people are flocking to doors of nursing school admission offices. Let me explain these points further.

The current nursing shortage is expected to increase to approximately 260,000 RNs by 2025 (Buerhaus, Auerbach, & Staiger, 2009). The reasons for the nursing shortage include a higher number of older hospitalized patients who need more care than did patients decades ago; a higher number of elderly people who have multiple chronic health conditions such as diabetes and heart disease; a growing array of work settings where nurses are employed other than hospitals such as home care, surgical centers, occupational health centers, etc.; and the high number of nurses who will reach retirement age between now and 2020 (AACN, 2010a, 2010b; Amos, 2005; HRSA, 2010). Obviously, where there is a high demand, there needs to be a high supply. Since nurses are currently, and will continue to be, in high demand, nurses have great job security for at least the next few decades. It is common for individuals who become nurses to retire as nurses, which indicates the longevity of nursing careers.

Nursing is considered a stable and financially rewarding career choice. Nurses enjoy very competitive pay and great benefits (see Chapter 1). Nurses willing to work nights and weekends or willing to work in specialties in high demand can make even more money. Nurses enjoy the usual full-time employment benefits of insurance and retirement plans, but they often also reap extra benefits such as assistance to pay for their education, flexible work schedules, and more weeks of vacation each year as compared to other professions. The stability of a career in nursing coupled with the favorable compensation package make entering the field of nursing appealing.

Another reason that people are attracted to a career in nursing is the rewarding nature of the work. A job satisfaction survey conducted by the U.S. Department of Health and Human Services Health Resources and Services Administration (HRSA, 2010) revealed that nurses really do love their jobs; 29.3% of the survey participants reported being extremely satisfied with their job and only 11.1% reported being dissatisfied with their job. The joy nurses find in their work strengthens the image of a desirable profession, which leads to more people wanting to become nurses, which results in more applications to nursing programs. After all, no one wants to spend thousands of dollars and hours on an education that leads to a career they will dislike.

Also, nurses have endless opportunities for working in different clinical specialties and settings. Nurses prepared at the BSN level are trained as generalists. This means that they learn a little bit about all types of nursing. Upon graduation, they can essentially apply for any entry-level nursing position, regardless of the setting or specialty. Then, after gaining some nursing experience and with a little networking, nurses are free to roam about and change from working in the cardiac unit, for example, to the intensive care unit, to the emergency department, to the outpatient clinic, and so on. Even further, nurses can choose to work in hospitals, but they can also work in long-term care and rehabilitation centers, specialty surgery centers, schools, for organizations like the American Red Cross, and more.

Given how much time the average person spends at work in his or her lifetime, it is so important to pursue a profession that you will love. A career in nursing has many appeals, ranging from high demand and job security to boundless opportunity for career development and advanced education. Keep in mind that there are many people who recognize the same tantalizing benefits of nursing as you do. Be honest with yourself and recognize the competition to earn a seat in a nursing class.

SEATS ARE GOING ... GOING ... GONE!

Now that you understand why there are so many nursing school applicants each year, let's explore why there are so few seats available in nursing schools. Schools of nursing face several very real constraints. Although schools are constantly implementing creative strategies and solutions, it would take nothing short of a magic wand to fix all of them immediately and permanently. The reasons for the limited capacity in nursing schools include a shortage of nursing faculty (teachers), a lack of clinical placements, budget limitations/cuts, a general lack of resources, and not enough preceptors for students.

Surveys conducted by both the National League for Nursing (NLN) and the AACN revealed that schools of nursing cited a shortage of nursing faculty as the number one reason they are not able to increase enrollment in their programs (Kaufman, 2010; AACN, 2010d). Several issues are fueling the faculty shortage. First, many nursing faculty positions now require a doctoral degree. There aren't enough nurses with doctoral degrees to fill the vacancies for teachers (AACN, 2010c). Specifically, there is a lack of nurses who are educationally qualified to teach. Another factor in the faculty shortage is that nurses can often make more money working in other types of nursing. For example, on average, teachers who have only a master's degree earn approximately 15% less per year than nurse practitioners who have a master's degree (AACN, 2010c). Schools find it difficult to recruit teachers from the competitive private sector. Nurses who go into teaching must look for other rewards beyond salary.

The lack of clinical placements is nearly as important as the shortage of nursing faculty (Kaufman, 2010; AACN, 2010c, 2010d). Clinical placements are the very crux of nursing education; they provide the real-life setting that nursing students need to practice their skills and learn how to deliver quality care to patients. Although many things can be imitated in laboratory settings with mannequins, real clinical experiences are where everything comes together for students. But, when several different schools in one city compete for the same clinical settings for their students, placements fill up quickly leaving no room for additional students. Every semester since I began working in nursing education, I have heard stories about clinical placements falling through at the last minute, leaving teachers scrambling and practically begging administrators of different health care settings to let their students come to their facilities. Finding enough clinical placements for all the students at *current* levels is one of the toughest jobs in the business. Increasing the number of students without a matching increase in clinical placement sites would simply be impossible.

And of course, schools today are also facing budget cuts, insufficient resources, and a lack of nurse preceptors for students (AACN, 2010a). In today's tough economic times, many colleges are forced to reduce overall budgets, slash spending, consolidate or eliminate expenses wherever possible, layoff teachers and/or staff, and enforce hiring freezes to stay in operation. Simply raising tuition rates on the students is not enough to make up for the budget shortfalls. Many nursing schools also lack other resources, such as classroom space and qualified preceptors needed to teach nursing students in the clinical setting.

Despite all this, you'll be encouraged to know that, somehow, schools are figuring out ways to let in a few more students. AACN (2010d) reported that the enrollment in BSN programs rose for the third straight year in 2010, up 3.6%. Schools of nursing have been able to expand their enrollments by implementing creative strategies to reduce the most critical issue: the nursing faculty shortage. For example, some schools allow nonnurses to teach certain courses, such as science courses. Other schools recruit nurses to go back to school to earn a graduate degree so that they will be qualified to teach, and other schools remove some of the financial restrictions usually placed on teachers who want to continue to work after they retire (AACN, 2005). Legislative strategies, such as federally funded programs that provide loan and scholarship support for nurses who go back to school, have also been used to increase the number of teachers. Schools have received other government grants to increase the number of laboratories and equipment so that schools may handle more students (AACN, 2010c).

ON YOUR MARK, GET SET, GO!

Now that you have a little background on why admission to nursing school is so competitive, it's time to focus your attention on two very key steps in your journey to becoming a nurse: (1) preparation for nursing school and (2) making your application stand out from the rest. My intention in this section is to give you practical, straightforward advice to guide you through these steps, with a focus on helping you submit a strong application that will rise to the top of the heap. Let's get started!

On Your Mark

The first step in preparing to enter nursing school requires *finding your mark*. In other words, you must be clear and confident in your goal to become a nurse. The nursing school application process is work-intensive, expensive, and time-consuming. The same could be said about nursing school. Therefore, you must be 100% convinced that nursing is the career you want. If possible, set up a nurse shadowing experience. Follow a nurse around for an afternoon and watch him in action. Watch him take vital signs, administer medication, confer with other members of the health care team, and listen to and talk to patients with care and attentiveness. If you have the opportunity, shadow several different nurses in different care settings (e.g., hospitals, assisted living centers, senior homes) and/or in different units (e.g., emergency, intensive care, oncology). This will widen your perspectives about the possibilities in nursing. Talk to the nurses about being a nurse. Ask them questions about their experiences in school, their work satisfaction, their complaints, their career plans, and the like. Try to envision yourself working as a nurse and doing what they do. Does this bring a smile to your face and raise your heart rate?

Health care–related work and volunteer experience is also a great way to help you reflect on whether or not nursing is right for you. Complete a certified nurse assistant (CNA) certification program at your local community college and work as a CNA. Or do something adventurous and volunteer with a team of nurses at health fairs, blood drives, or free medical clinics. Spend time at your local senior center visiting with the residents and observing the work of their caregivers. Volunteer at an organization like the American Red Cross and witness how health care professionals spring into action.

After you've had the chance to spend a few days in the life of a nurse, it's important that you take time for in-depth personal reflection about what you observed, how it made you feel, what excited you about it, and what questions it raised for you. Ask yourself if nursing is truly the right path for you. If all signs say "yes," your next reflection should focus on how nursing school will mesh with the realities of your life. Ask yourself if it is the right time for you to start school in terms of where you are on your career path, the dynamics of your family life, and your financial state. Do you have a support system in place to encourage you through the heights of your stress? Can people help with childcare or even share the load of household duties while you're in school? Nursing school is inherently challenging and difficult. Are you ready to buckle-down and work like you've never worked before? Do you have a sufficient financial aid package or a realistic plan for paying for your education? These are the types of questions you must ask yourself, and answer honestly.

After you've seen nursing with your own eyes, gained some work and/ or volunteer experience in health care, and taken time for personal reflection, you should feel confident in your decision to pursue a nursing career. Having confidence in your decision, you will be ready to tackle the application process for nursing school with the attention and effort it requires and deserves. You should plan to bring a little toughness and a competitive spirit to "get set," the next step in becoming nurse.

Get Set

You've found your mark, so now it's time to think about the application process for nursing school. My advice is to respect the process and take it seriously. This is not the time to procrastinate, slack-off, make assumptions, or ill-prepare. If you really want to be a nurse, then prepare yourself to work hard not only in nursing school, but also on the steps it takes to get there. Be aware that it may take you a year or more to complete the "get set" step, so be patient and stick with it.

Start with academics. All nursing school admission committees want to see that you have worked hard in school and have been successful. They often require that you complete a specific list of prerequisite (required) courses as part of the application process. The list of prerequisite courses can vary widely, depending on what type of program you are applying to (e.g., associate's, bachelor's, accelerated bachelor's, second-degree, direct-entry master's) and at what type of institution (e.g., private university, religious school, public college, community college). What remains the same across all program types and institutions, however, is that each application review committee expects you to do *really* well in your coursework. And you need to do *really* well in *all* of your courses, not just in your prerequisite courses.

Nursing schools often set a minimum cumulative (total) GPA requirement for admission. The important thing to understand here is that your cumulative GPA is with you for life. There is no way to go back and change it. So, that history course you earned a D in during your freshman year because you slept through your alarm clock on final exam day is factored into your

GPA, just like that A you received in advanced calculus. If you attended several different schools, keep in mind that the nursing school you are applying to may average all of the cumulative GPAs together, factoring in how many credits you completed at each school. For example, if your cumulative GPA was a 3.00 after 100 credits at School A and your cumulative GPA at School B was a 2.00 but only after 3 credits (1 class), your overall cumulative GPA would be a 2.97. Even if you attended School B a long time ago, it is still part of the cumulative GPA calculation. In this case, if the minimum admission requirement for the nursing school was 3.00, you would not meet it. But don't get discouraged; it works the other way, too! Say that you're a tenth of a grade point away from meeting a school's cumulative GPA minimum. Enroll in some courses that would be beneficial to you in nursing school, such as writing, computer skills, or speech. Earn top grades in these new classes, and watch your overall cumulative GPA climb upward.

In addition to a cumulative GPA minimum, it is common for nursing schools to set another type of GPA minimum, such as a GPA based only on the prerequisite science courses. This can be very important, since the best predictor of success in nursing school is science GPA (Wolkowitz & Kelley, 2010). It follows then, that admission committees often consider the science GPA to be the most important admission factor. Review your transcripts. If you received a C+ or below in any of the required prerequisite science courses, I strongly encourage you to re-take them for a better grade. The harsh truth is that if your science GPA is low, you may never be given serious consideration, even if the rest of your application is amazing. On the other hand, an excellent science GPA may give your file the review it may otherwise not have had. For example, say you are applying to a school and your cumulative GPA isn't very strong, but you have a science GPA of a perfect 4.00. In this instance, your science GPA is a golden opportunity. Even if your cumulative GPA falls short of the minimum requirement, a very high science GPA may still bring attention to your file. The bottomline then is to study hard, focus on your prerequisite courses, especially the science courses, and do your very best to earn high grades.

Another piece of the "getting set" step you'll likely encounter is the requirement of a standardized test. If you are applying to a university right out of high school, you will probably be required to take either the Scholastic Aptitude Test (SAT) or the American College Test (ACT). If you are applying to an associate's or bachelor's degree in nursing program, you may be required to take another test that is specific to nursing, such as the Assessment Technology Institute's Test of Essential Academic Skills. This test has sections in science, math, reading, and English. Scores on the science and reading sections have been shown to predict early success in nursing school (Wolkowitz & Kelley, 2010). Applicants to direct-entry master's programs are usually asked to take the Graduate Record Examination (GRE), which is thought to predict success in graduate-level courses. Whichever test the nursing school requires for admission, be sure to take it seriously by studying ahead of time and taking the test well in advance of the application deadline. For each test, there are resources available to help you study. Download the study guides and software programs, take a preparation class, or buy preparation books. Schedule time every day or few days to study for the test. Stick to your schedule; don't skip your study time. When you feel ready, take the test. I recommend scheduling your test date approximately 8 weeks prior to the application deadline. This allows plenty of time for your scores to be processed and sent to the school. It also allows enough time for you to retake the test for a better score, if necessary. It is quite common, and perfectly acceptable, to take the test more than once. Usually, students improve their scores the second time around.

Deciding on which schools to apply to

There are many options and factors to consider in deciding which colleges and program types to apply to. First, there are various nursing program types and degree options available (see Table 4.1). You can easily narrow down your options by researching the minimum level of education (e.g., high school, bachelor's degree) required for entry. For example, let's say you are interested in a nursing baccalaureate program. One BSN program may list a high-school diploma as the minimum education requirement. Another BSN program for transfer students may require a minimum of 60 semester hours of college credit. A direct-entry master's program will require a bachelor's degree in a nonnursing field as the minimum education requirement. If you won't have a college degree when you enter nursing school, but you have some college credit already, then your only option of these three schools is the BSN transfer program. You've efficiently eliminated two options from your list!

After you have figured out what type of program you are eligible to apply to, create a list of schools that interest you that offer this program. Research each of the schools in terms of acceptance rates, class size, format, length, cost, quality, quality of the teachers, accreditation status, NCLEX-RN® (nurse licensure exam) pass rates, and the school's mission and reputation. I suggest building a table that will help you easily compare the pros and cons of each school. Much of this information is available on school websites

TABLE 4.1   Nursing Program Options

PROGRAM TYPE	APPROXIMATE LENGTH	MINIMUM EDUCATION REQUIREMENT
Associate Degree in Nursing (ADN)	2–3 years	High school diploma or GED
Traditional Bachelor of Science in Nursing Degree (BSN)	4 years	High school diploma or GED
Transfer BSN	1.5–3 years	College credit (number of credits required varies)
Accelerated BSN	1–1.5 years	Bachelor's degree in a non-nursing major
Direct Entry Master's (DEM) or Entry Level Master's Degree (ELM)	2–6 years	Bachelor's degree in a non-nursing major

and in information packets. While program counselors are usually available to offer assistance and answer questions, it is always appreciated if you do some research on your own. This way, you will come prepared with specific questions. In addition to information on websites or from counselors, you can learn more from information nights or visitation days. At these events, schools invite prospective students to campus for a presentation about the details of the program. You can arrange a tour of campus to feel the campus vibe, see the facilities, and perhaps even meet teachers or students. Speaking of students, find a way to connect with a current student or graduate to hear his/her testimonial about the program. Students will tell you what it's *really* like to be a nursing student at that program.

After gathering your information, carefully evaluate whether any of the schools on your list should be removed. For example, if a program has a history of low NCLEX-RN pass rates or charges tuition rates that are out of your range, or the school schedule doesn't accommodate your family or work schedule, then don't waste your time applying to it. Trying to make a poorly fit school fit your life is not worth the stress you will endure.

Staying organized

Sometimes it seems like nursing school applicants have to go through a difficult maze just to get everything completed correctly and on time. Every school has its own application deadlines, checklists, required forms, essay prompts, and prerequisite courses. Differences among schools can be confusing and overwhelming; therefore, be meticulous. Write down and double check the application deadlines, admission requirements, and prerequisite lists at each of the schools you're interested in applying to. This advice cannot be overstated.

Imagine this scenario: You have a 4.00 science GPA and a strong essay. You meet the minimum entrance exam requirements, but one of your college transcripts arrives in the mail one day *after* the application deadline. Or, imagine that you scored in the top 2% on the entrance exam, but there was a glitch in the reporting system and your report never made it to the admission office. At most schools, both of these situations would mean your application file wouldn't even be reviewed. This could shatter your chance of starting nursing school on time. Don't let this happen to you! I suggest you track the many moving parts involved in applying to several different nursing schools at the same time by making a table. This table should include the name of each school you will apply to on different rows. In columns, enter each of these categories:

- Application deadline
- Application fee, including acceptable methods of payment
- Mailing address, phone number, fax number, and email address of the office/department your application needs to be submitted to
- Admission counselor contact information
- School and/or program web address
- Admission requirements, including minimum GPAs and/or test scores
- A list of prerequisite courses, along with your progress/plan to complete them

Keep this table updated and make notes on it about your progress. Keep track of all communication you have with people at the school. Keep copies of emails and letters. These provide documentation in case there are any questions about your status. Meet with an admission counselor and seek his/her advice about how to ensure that the application process goes smoothly for you. Admission professionals often have special insider tips to share. Basically, do whatever you can to keep yourself organized and on the right track toward completing each of your applications on time.

GO!

OK, now it's to time to prepare those application packets. It's time to "Go!" In this section, review my practical tips on how to make your application stand out from the rest by following these key points:

- Make sure your application actually gets reviewed
- Never leave an application question blank
- Get quality recommendation letters
- I know it's tempting, but resist essay templates!
- Just because it isn't required doesn't meet you can't or shouldn't submit it.
- If there is something in your academic history that needs explaining then get to it!
- Shamelessly toot your own horn

First things first: make sure your application actually gets reviewed. I know it seems like I am stating the obvious here, but I can't tell you the number of times I have had to explain to applicants that their application was never reviewed because just one piece of their file was not received by the deadline. It's heartbreaking news to deliver and to hear. Again, double- and triple-check with admission offices to ensure that the items you send are received and placed in your application file. Although admission offices are extremely busy around deadline time, don't worry about bothering anyone or being a pest. Call, email, or do whatever it takes to make sure that your file is completed on time. Other things you can do to make sure your file is eligible to review are:

- *Take the required entrance exam early and be sure to request that your official report be sent to the appropriate department.* Count back about 8 weeks from the application deadline and set that as your goal for taking the exam. If the testing center will require a school or department code, make sure you have that information at your fingertips when you register. *Note: You might want to request that two or three official copies be sent to you as well. Keep them sealed and in a safe place in case you need them in the future or need to provide an additional copy.*
- *Request that your official school transcript(s) be sent ASAP.* For some reason, transcripts are like socks in a dryer—they just seem to disappear! Remove this potential obstacle and make your transcript requests early so that you could request another copy if your original request doesn't

make it. Keep common school breaks (e.g., spring break, winter break) and holidays in mind since admission offices might be closed and plan accordingly.

■ *Be diligent when gathering recommendation letters*. People are busy. Don't assume that one email to your supporter is enough. Be sure to check-in with your letter writers often and provide any information that would be helpful to them.

Second, never leave an application question blank. Given the volume of applicants, you may think there is no way that a review committee is actually going to read every item on every application. Thinking this way may guarantee your rejection letter. Consider this example:

> It's the final day of making admission decisions for a nursing school review committee. Stephen and Adam are two applicants who are almost identical in terms of numerical measures—they have 3.82 and 3.85 science GPAs, have 3.78 and 3.80 cumulative GPAs, and the exact same standardized test scores. The review committee only has one more seat available and they need a tie-breaker. What makes the review committee send Stephen an acceptance letter instead of Adam? Stephen answered each of the application questions thoroughly with no grammatical errors. He wove-in how the school's mission matches his own personal set of values and beliefs. In contrast, Adam didn't bother to answer the open-ended questions on the application. He only answered the required fields on the on-line application.

If you were in the review committee's position, wouldn't you have made the same decision to accept Stephen and not Adam?

Not only is it important to fill in every field, it is important to demonstrate that you are a match with the institution and program. Look up the school's mission and vision. You can find these on their website or information materials. Also, research the school's reputation, any special awards or recognition the school has received, and recent headlines about the school in local newspapers. Try to weave this information into your answers or essay on the application. This will show the review committee that you are impressed with their school and are determined to enroll. After all, reviewers want to accept students who really want to be there, not just students who are likely to succeed.

Third, get *quality* recommendation letters. In short, choose your supporters wisely. Don't have a nurse you've only shadowed once write you a letter just because he is an RN. Sure, reviewers admire letters written by health care professionals, but if the person barely knows you, how can he write you a quality letter? Instead, choose individuals who know you well, who will take the time to write you a thoughtful letter. Ideally, choose supporters who know a bit about the program and/or school you are applying to. Think about who you know that can speak to your likelihood of success in nursing school, your passion for the profession, your work ethic and professionalism, and your leadership skills. Try to choose a few different supporters so that each of them can provide insight into a different piece of you. For example, pick a science teacher to provide insight to your academic ability, a health care professional to provide insight to your passion for nursing, and a supervisor to provide insight to your professionalism. Think of recommendation letters as a window into who you are as a student, a professional, and a person. Make sure the review committee will like what they see in your recommendation letters. Another way to get quality recommendation letters is to prepare the writers. Give each person a prestamped, preaddressed envelope, a bulleted list of the topics you would like them to discuss in the letter, your resume, and any school forms they need to fill out; and maybe throw in a chocolate bar or two as a token of your appreciation! Your letter writers will be impressed by your preparedness and will appreciate that they do not have to dig for the details. In turn, this will help you get better letters and a stronger application file.

Fourth, I know it's tempting, but resist using templates for your essay! Don't think you can pull one over on the nursing school admission teams by submitting the same essay to every school you apply to. Believe me, they'll catch on to you. The essay is not the place to take shortcuts; it is often the only way that review committees can get to know who you are as a person. Consider the essay your time to shine. Different schools have different essay prompts, word requirements, and page limits for the essays, so using the same essay for each school won't work. Sure, you can use the same basic information for each essay, but you need to tailor each essay to each school. Write each essay with a fresh attitude and equal rigor. Make it appear to the reviewers that you are applying only to their school and no other.

Fifth, just because a school doesn't require something doesn't mean you can't or shouldn't submit it. Some schools require essays or personal statements, recommendation letters, and resumes while others may require only some of these items. Whatever the case, know that it can only help your chances of acceptance if you submit supplemental information that might make you appear to be a stronger applicant. The more information you provide, the more detailed the picture the reviewers have of you. When you are compared against hundreds of other applicants, whatever you can submit to show your uniqueness, higher qualifications, and solid understanding of and passion for nursing will increase your chances of receiving an admission offer. Consider writing a summary of your volunteer work, international, and/or health care–related experience. Submit a copy of your CNA license, awards you received, or other certifications you've earned. If the application requires one recommendation letter, send three letters instead. Provide a sample of your scholarly writing or a copy of a presentation you delivered. Get creative and fill up your file!

Sixth, if there is something in your academic history that needs explaining, then do so. Admissions professionals understand that personal tragedies, medical illnesses, and other life happenings can have a negative effect on academic performance. They also realize that a difficult experience shouldn't haunt you for the rest of your life and prevent you from becoming a nurse. If you feel that a grade, series of grades, or entrance exam score does not reflect your true academic ability, I recommend that you explain it by submitting a statement with your application. Don't cross your fingers and hope that the reviewers don't notice it. For instance, if a loved one passed away during Spring semester of your sophomore year and your transcript has a string of low grades during that time, submit an attachment that explains your relationship to the loved one and how the grief from their passing affected you emotionally and academically. Or perhaps you are an older student who first went to college 15 years ago and are now applying to a second-degree program. You thought it would be exciting to go to a school far away from home. However, you quickly grew to miss your family and friends and had a tough time transitioning to college life. You ended your first semester of college with a 2.27 GPA. After you transferred to a college closer to home, your grades shot up to a 3.6 average GPA. It would be helpful for the review committee to find an attachment in your application file that explains the low GPA during your first semester of college. Think about the possibility that a review committee could be down to their very last admission decision and it's between you and another applicant; having an explanation for something negative in your file could tip the scales in your favor.

Eight, shamelessly toot your own horn. It makes some people uncomfortable to brag about their accomplishments and draw attention to their unique experiences, talents, and abilities. If that's the case for you, then accept the fact that applying to nursing school is going to make you feel a bit uneasy. Think about your application like a resume. Resumes are meant to highlight all the ways in which you are a perfect candidate for the job. Likewise, when applying to nursing school, you need to show why *you* are the most deserving of all applicants for a seat in the school's nursing program. There may never be a more important time for you to gloat and brag about yourself. This is not the time to minimize your greatness. Here are some examples of experiences you should definitely make evident in your application file, if they apply to you:

- Ability to speak a foreign language
- International experience, especially if it is health care–related
- Volunteer experience, especially if it is health care–related
- Health care–related certifications and/or work experience
- Involvement in clubs, organizations, and/or student government, especially if you held leadership positions
- Any professional experience in areas such as business, policy, informatics, and education, with your thoughts of how this experience will make you a better nurse
- Awards and honors earned in the community, professional, and/or educational setting
- Being the first one in your family to attend college
- Overcoming a significant challenge (e.g., poverty, abuse, addiction, immigration from a foreign country)

Basically, think of all the ways you are different from other applicants. Explain how these differences give you an advantage over other potential students. There are many ways to weave your accomplishments throughout your application. Your essay is a perfect place to tell your story that will make you stand above all others. Another place to highlight your achievements is in your resume. In addition, you might want to consider writing a separate summary of your work and/or volunteer experience and how it has prepared you for nursing. Lastly, you can submit copies of awards and certificates you have received. By now, I'm sure you catch my drift—shine the spotlight on yourself.

SUMMARY

I've given you a lot of information! I have explained why there are so many nursing school applicants and so few seats available for students. I have offered practical advice to help you prepare for nursing school and make your application stand out. Nursing is a hot career choice today due to nursing's job security, good salaries, endless opportunities, and the rewarding nature of working as a nurse. However, nursing schools face very real constraints that prevent them from expanding enrollment. The most significant constraints are shortage of nursing faculty and lack of sites to place students for their clinical experiences. With all these competing forces at play, it is likely that nursing school admissions will remain highly competitive for the foreseeable future. I have presented a number of tips to help you. While I believe they are *all* important, here are six tips that summarize my advice to you:

1. Be really sure that nursing is the right career choice for you.
2. Do your research about nursing, nursing schools, and application requirements.
3. Do your very best in science courses.
4. Essays and application questions allow an admission committee to get to know you. Take these essays and questions seriously; spend time on them and openly brag about yourself.
5. Always assume that the last admission decision for a committee is going to be between you and someone else. Fill your file with extra information that will serve as the tie-breaker.
6. And finally, good luck! Visualize success for yourself, and make it happen!

REFERENCES

American Association of Colleges of Nursing. (2005). *Faculty shortages in baccalaureate and graduate programs: Scope of the problem and strategies for expanding the supply*. Retrieved from http://www.aacn.nche.edu/Publications/WhitePapers/FacultyShortages.htm

American Association of Colleges of Nursing. (2010a). *The future of higher education in nursing: 2010 annual report*. Retrieved from http://www.aacn.nche.edu/media/pdf/AnnualReport10.pdf

American Association of Colleges of Nursing. (2010b). *Nursing shortage* [Fact sheet]. Retrieved from http://www.aacn.nche.edu/media/FactSheets/NursingShortage.htm

American Association of Colleges of Nursing. (2010c). *Addressing the nursing shortage: A focus on nurse faculty.* Retrieved from http://www.aacn.nche.edu/Government/pdf/NrsShrtgStrats.pdf

American Association of Colleges of Nursing. (2010d). *Amid calls for more highly educated nurses, new AACN data shows impressive growth in doctoral nursing programs.* Retrieved from http://www.aacn.nche.edu/media/newsreleases/2010/enrollchanges.html

American Association of Colleges of Nursing. (2012). *New AACN data show an enrollment surge in baccalaureate and graduate programs amid calls for more highly educated nurses.* Retrieved from http://www.aacn.nche.edu/news/articles/2012/enrollment-data

Amos, L.K. (2005). *Baccalaureate nursing programs.* Retrieved from http://www.aacn.nche.edu/Education/nurse_ed_BSNArticle.htm.

Buerhaus, P. I., Auerbach, D. I. & Staiger, D. O. (2009, July/August). The recent surge in nursing employment: causes and implications. *Health Affairs, 28*(4), 657–668.

Human Resources and Services Administration (HRSA). (2010, March). *The registered nurse population: Initial findings from the 2008 national sample survey of registered nurses.* Retrieved from http://bhpr.hrsa.gov/healthworkforce/rnsurvey/2008/nssrn2008.pdf

Kaufman, K.A. (2010, May/June). Findings from the annual survey of schools of nursing academic year 2008–2009: Students are increasingly diverse but lack of educational capacity still stymies enrollment growth. *Nursing Education Perspectives, 31*(3), 196–197.

Wolkowitz, A. A. & Kelley, J. A. (2010). *Academic predictors of success in a nursing program. Journal of Nursing Education, 49*(9), 498–503.

FIVE

How to Avoid Getting Voted Off the Island: How to Survive Nursing School

Congratulations! All your hard work has paid off. You are now enrolled in a nursing program. If you're like most entering students, you are excited but a little nervous. You've heard that nursing school is difficult. You know that you're usually up to a challenge, but did you bite off more than you can chew this time? Is the talk you've heard just stuff to get you spooked? Will you really fit in? Is nursing school going to turn out the way you thought?

Every student's journey in nursing school is different, but most journeys have some similarities. My own journey was no exception. I was so excited to get started. I remember the first day of my class like it was yesterday. I remember looking around the room, my eyes scanning my new classmates. I remember wanting to find someone who might become a study partner, a confidante, a new friend, but nobody looked like someone I would naturally hang out with. I remember getting nervous, but that didn't last too long. I knew I would eventually make new friends. Looking back now, I realize that I was completely unprepared for what would lie ahead. Although I had been in college for several years and received very good grades, nursing school was different. My previous study habits, the amount of time I usually devoted to homework, and my general attitude toward school all proved to be a misfit to what was needed in nursing school. Like most students, I muddled though my courses and eventually finished. Obviously, muddling through does not result in an ideal education. I did OK, but did not take advantage of all the learning opportunities that were available to me at that time. I finished nursing school with only a few bumps and bruises. Some students don't fare so well; they fall by the wayside and never receive their nursing degrees. Sadly, many of these students could have been successful with a little more foresight, and possibly, with a little more self-discipline.

Nursing school poses many challenges that may make the student journey difficult. Another term for these challenges is *barriers*. If ignored, barriers may prevent you from finishing nursing school. But don't worry. If you know the common barriers as you start nursing school, you can use strategies to jump over the barriers if they come your way. In some ways, you can think of nursing school as *Survivor*, the popular television reality show. Knowing which barriers might come your way and how to work around those barriers will do much in preventing you from getting "voted off the island." In other words, minimizing the potential harm from barriers will help you be more successful and prevent you from getting failing grades that will direct you to the exit doors. In this chapter, I'll discuss the common barriers experienced by most nursing students, where these barriers come from, and how to overcome these barriers. Also, I'll give special attention to the unique barriers experienced by men. This chapter should make you sit up and take notice. Clearly, you'll never become a nurse if you don't make it through nursing school first. However, to become a great nurse, you'll need to create the best school experience possible and develop habits of life-long learning that will serve you well as you launch your career.

WHY IS NURSING SCHOOL SO TOUGH?

As a professor and academic advisor, students ask me this question often. Some students find themselves floundering after taking only a few nursing courses. Past success strategies no longer seem to work. The courses are sometimes much harder than expected. There are pages and pages of complex reading every night. The amount of time to prepare for clinical experiences is greater than had been planned. Family time and other obligations seem to get pushed aside. The levels of stress and anxiety seem to mount week-by-week until something has to give. Does nursing school really have to be this tough? The short answer is "yes"; your future and the well-being of your future patients require that nursing school prepares you to be the best nurse possible.

I received a very different education when I started nursing school in the early 1980s than the education students have today. The focus of my education was to learn how to *do*, not to learn *why* or *how*. For example, I took anatomy and physiology. In this class, I learned the body parts and how they functioned at a basic level. In the lab, I learned that I should elevate the feet of a patient who has swollen ankles. I was never taught to connect the two: that elevating the feet helps water flow back into the veins, thus reducing the swollen ankles. I was simply told that elevating the feet would reduce swelling, and that I should do this because it works. Enough said! Further, the impression I had was that the same nursing action should be given to every patient who had the same problem. So, for all my patients with swollen ankles, I should elevate their feet. If I had been challenged to connect physiology with the nursing action, I would have learned that elevating the feet of someone with very swollen ankles without a method to remove the excess water may, in fact, harm the patient's heart. Learning only what to do creates nurses who treat every problem the same way. These kinds of nurses don't think about what makes every patient and every problem different. Worse, nurses taught this way often become dependent on others to tell them what to do. These nurses have poor problem-solving skills. These nurses could be dangerous if they can't think through what they need to do in different situations, unless they update and deepen their knowledge.

Today, we demand much more of our nurses. Scientific discoveries and technological breakthroughs have increased the knowledge required of nurses. Nurses must understand incredibly complex patient conditions embedded in incredibly complex systems of care. In addition, nurses must assume leadership for teams of health professionals because nurses have the most contact with patients (Crowell, 2011; Institute of Medicine [IOM], 2011). Nurses must coordinate all the pieces of a patient's health care so that goals are met, while at the same time, serve as the caring human face in an often faceless and confusing health care system. There is so much more to learn in school than was required of me, yet students must finish school in the same amount of time. It's no wonder school is so tough!

The amount students must learn today has re-ignited the entry-to-practice debate. For decades, American nurse leaders have argued about the minimum level of education required to be a nurse. This argument has never been resolved. Today, students may become licensed as a nurse after earning an associate's degree, a diploma (hospital-based school), a bachelor's degree, or even a master's degree. However, a few well-publicized studies suggest that having a higher degree, at least a bachelor's degree, seems to matter. Some patients who have nurses with this level of education do better (Kendall-Gallagher, Aiken, Sloane, & Cimiotti, 2011; Aiken, Clarke, Cheung, Sloane, & Silber, 2003). Other nations, such as Canada, Australia, and the United Kingdom, have moved to the bachelor's degree as the minimum requirement for nurses (Rheaume, 2003). American nurse leaders have been slower to move. In 2011, the Tri-Council for Nursing (a body of four national nursing organizations concerned about education and the nursing profession) issued a statement that read, in part, "These [nursing] competencies require increased education at all levels....Without a more educated nursing workforce, the nation's health will be further at risk" (American Association of Colleges of Nursing, 2011, para. 2). The Tri-Council did not push for a minimum education level for nurses; instead, they asked that all parties work together to help nurses advance their education. The IOM was bolder. In their *Future of Nursing* report (IOM, 2011), this group of experts declared that the profession needs more nurses who have bachelor's degrees and higher. They recommended that nurses who earn an associate's degree should obtain their bachelor's degrees early in their careers if they are to be the nurses needed in health care today. Some employers stipulate that nurses earn their bachelor's degrees within five years after being hired if they do not already have this degree.

Personally, I wonder how students can learn so much in such a short period of time. I see students working harder than ever before. The typical four years to earn a bachelor's degree is not enough. Where I teach now, we require students to come to summer school at least once. Many students come to school for several summers so that they can graduate on time. The four-year bachelor's degree often now takes five school-years to complete. Even with this extra time, most students struggle to learn everything we expect. As we move into the future, science and technology will only become more advanced. Nurses will have to catch up. I would not be surprised that, someday, we will consider the master's degree as the required minimum for nurses.

Nursing teachers have had to change too. With many scientific and tech-nological advances, teachers have had to increase their own knowledge of the changing health care environment. Teachers are now asked to teach more complicated subjects in a shorter amount of time. Teachers have to learn new ways to infuse technology into classrooms to make content come alive and stimulate learning. In this information age, teachers must now sort through mountains of information and determine which information should be used and which information should be set aside. Today, it's no longer acceptable for teachers to simply have their students read and recite the material. Today, teachers must expect students to explain, analyze, problem-solve, and inno-vate. In order for this to happen, students must take greater ownership for their own learning. Students are asked to do more homework, more inde-pendent study, and spend more time collaborating with other classmates on group projects. When I think back to my own days as a nursing student, I realize that I received the lowest level of an education by today's standards. And nursing school seemed tough back then!

With so much to learn in so little time, it's easy to see how school can be stressful. Without proper supports, the stress might become overwhelming and students might drop out, or worse, fail nursing school. Leaving school before finishing is called *attrition*. Attrition has worried nurse teachers for some time. After all, if students don't finish school, then we have fewer stu-dents becoming nurses and joining the nurse workforce. The national rates for attrition from nursing school are unknown since there is disagreement on how to define attrition. For example, some students leave school for a while and then re-enter and finish at a later date. Sometimes these stu-dents are counted with those who drop out of school; sometimes they are not. To address the problem, the British government developed a common definition of attrition and is now requiring schools to have attrition rates less than 13% (Deary, Watson, & Hogston, 2003). This will challenge some schools since average attrition rates in the United Kingdom range from 6% to 24% depending upon the location (Pryjmachuk, Easton, & Littlewood, 2008; Urwin et al., 2010).

In the United States, no standard definition for attrition is available. Schools may vary in how they calculate attrition rates and report them to the U.S. Department of Education. The National League for Nursing (2011a) esti-mated U.S. attrition rates at about 12–25% in 2006, depending upon the type of nursing program (e.g., baccalaureate vs. diploma programs). Although these rates are better than the attrition rates for college students in gen-eral (U.S. Department of Education, 2011), each student that leaves nursing school takes up a precious spot that could have been used by another stu-dent who may have finished. Of greater importance to you, leaving school before graduation is disappointing considering all the hard work and money you invested in becoming a nurse.

The attrition rate for male nursing students is probably higher than the rate for female nursing students. Unfortunately, there are no readily available national statistics on how likely men are to leave nursing school. The only data available are from individual schools. Sprouse (1996) claimed that about 50% of male students drop out or fail nursing school. Wilson (2005) reported that the attrition rate for men at the nursing school he studied was 55.5%. At a school I examined, men were six times more likely to fail a nursing course than were women. Higher failure or drop-out rates for male students were reported in Britain and Northern Ireland as well (Pryjmachuk, Easton, & Littlewood, 2008; McLaughlin, Muldoon, & Moutray, 2010; Mulholland, Anionwu, Atkins, Tappern, & Franks, 2008; White, Williams, & Green, 1999). This information suggests that either men face more challenges in nursing school than do women, that nursing schools are failing at meeting the needs of male students, or both. Don't worry, many men do quite well in nursing school, but something is different for male nursing students. First, let's look at the barriers that all students might face; then I'll focus on barriers that are unique to men.

GENERAL NURSING SCHOOL BARRIERS

Much has been written about barriers faced by nursing students. Some of these barriers have changed over time, as nursing schools and education practices have changed. Also, each student experiences barriers differently. For example, some students struggle with juggling family obligations and homework; others juggle these easily. How any one barrier may affect you can't be predicted with any certainty; you will have to reflect on your own personal situation and preferences, as well as the common practices seen at your school in order to determine which barriers pose the greatest risk to your success. Urwin et al. (2010) stated that most students leave school for multiple reasons, so several barriers usually work together to threaten your success. In order to understand these barriers, these authors examined articles published between 1950 and 2009. They organized barriers into three categories: those caused by (a) individual student factors, (b) school factors, and (c) political-professional factors.

Barriers Caused by Individual Student Factors

Academic preparation
In Chapter 4, Stacey Boatright talks about the importance of academic preparation (good grades) in getting into nursing school, especially preparation in science courses. But academic preparation also predicts success in finishing nursing school. In one study looking at over 1,100 British nursing students, overall academic preparation was one of the strongest predictors for completing nursing school (Pryjmachuk, Easton, & Littlewood, 2008). This finding confirmed the same results from earlier British studies (Houltram, 1996; Kevern, Rickett, & Webb, 1999), a study from Canada (Wong & Wong, 1999), and from multiple American studies (Campbell & Dickson, 1996; Fowles, 1992; Higgins, 2005; Horns, O'Sullivan, & Goodman, 1991; Lewis & Lewis, 2000). But all types of academic preparation are not the same; good grades in science classes were especially important in finishing nursing school (Lewis & Lewis, 2000; Wong & Wong, 1999). Furthermore, good science preparation was the strongest predictor of *early* success in nursing school as well (Potolsky, Cohen, & Saylor, 2003; Wolkowitz & Kelley, 2010).

An important barrier faced by some students is having poor academic skills before starting nursing school that are then carried on into their nursing classes. I see this barrier in some of my own students. I have taught pathophysiology for a number of years. This course is probably the most difficult course in the nursing program, but it is one of the most important. In this course, students learn about changes in the body that lead to illness and disease. They also learn why these changes lead to signs and symptoms they will find in their future patients. Every semester, a handful of students really struggle in this course. There are a number of reasons for their struggles, but often I find out that these students barely made it through anatomy and physiology (courses in which they learn how the body works when it is healthy). Many of these students also struggled in their other science courses. It's difficult to learn new material in nursing school when you haven't first mastered material from courses you took in the past. Specifically, without knowing how the body works when it is healthy, you will have trouble understanding how the body works when it is unhealthy. Students who come to nursing school with poor science backgrounds will find nursing school very tough from the very start. These students may never recover and may never graduate.

Study habits. Poor academic preparation often is caused by poor study habits. Frequently, students develop poor study habits before starting nursing school and continue to use them once they have started their nursing classes. Sometimes bad habits are not severe enough to cause a student to fail at first. However, as students move ahead, the nursing classes become more difficult, and poor study habits will eventually lead to failing grades. Some students refuse to accept that their failure is due to their poor study habits. Since these habits did not cause them to fail a class in the past, these students assume that their failure is due, instead, to unfair teachers, excessive homework, or one of many other excuses. However, what should be obvious is that the usual study habits aren't working anymore. Students must take ownership of their study habits and change habits that aren't helpful. Common types of poor study habits I see include poor time management and over-reliance on memorization.

Poor time management, specifically not allowing enough time for studying, is common among students. Part of the problem here is that many beginning nursing students underestimate the amount of time it takes to complete all their homework and prepare for classes and clinical experiences. It's easy to understand why this problem occurs. Many students figure out how much time it takes to study in their prenursing classes. They get a general feel for how long it takes to read the books, write papers, and prepare for exams. Once this is learned, many students fill the rest of their schedules with other activities, such as family time, work, or recreation. Upon entering nursing school, sometimes this time schedule no longer works. Nursing school often requires time commitments that are not always reflected on student course schedules. This means that a three-credit nursing class may need more homework time than a three-credit history class. For example, the time needed to prepare for clinical experiences can be great and is not always counted in the credit hours listed for the class. In addition, students may have to travel across town to *attend* certain clinical experiences. The commute time may be much longer than the time it takes to commute to school. In many nursing courses, there are usually more required pages to read than in many prenursing classes. In one study, it was reported that less than half of the nursing students completed their homework for their pathophysiology class (Salamonson, Andrew, & Everett, 2009). Another study found only 11% of nursing students reporting that they completed the assigned readings on time (Purdue, 2009). In this same study, students reported that they spent between 6 and 10 hours a week doing homework. This may be far short of what is needed. Although there is no magic number for the right amount to spend on homework, I have seen recommendations that students should be expected to spend between 2 and 4 hours per week on homework for every scheduled hour of class. For a typical nursing student taking 12 credit hours in a semester, that would equal between *24 and 48 hours of homework per week*. This is why I tell students that being a full-time student is the same as having a full-time, 40-hour-per-week job. Spending 10 hours per week on homework will not be enough for most students to earn good grades.

However, it isn't just the *amount* of time spent on homework that is important. The *quality* of the time spent is also important. Plant, Ericsson, Hill, and Asberg (2005) reported that increased study time only leads to better grades if the quality of the study time is considered. Obviously, studying in a setting that is noisy or distracting does not lead to improved learning. Ramdass and Zimmerman (2011) reported that many studies suggested that the ability to reduce distractions during studying is important in making study time effective.

Another poor study habit is an overreliance on memorization. Magnussen (2001) stated that researchers believe that memorization only provides surface learning in which students learn information only as it is presented by the teacher or in a book. Hoffman (2008) pointed out that there is just too much health and nursing information to memorize, and what is memorized today may be out-of-date tomorrow. This reality hits many students hard. Some students throw up their hands in frustration when their memorization habits no longer work for them. They assume that if there is too much to memorize, then the teacher has put too much information in the class.

Memorized knowledge cannot be applied to real-life nursing situations in which the nurse must solve complex situations that are different from patient to patient. In effect, memorization does not foster *critical thinking*. Critical thinking has been defined in many different ways, but Riddell (2007) credited Stephen Brookfield, an expert on teaching, on setting the groundwork for the most common definitions of critical thinking. Brookfield noted that critical thinking requires a person to examine the big picture of a situation, analyze assumptions, and explore and imagine alternative solutions to problems. Critical thinking forces you to reflect on what you are doing and challenge the assumption that there is one right answer to every situation. Since today's health care environment requires nurses to be critical thinkers (Riddell), teachers have started to use classroom activities that promote active learning, which in turn will develop critical thinking skills (Magnussen, 2001; Popkess & McDaniel, 2011). Instead of the old-fashioned approach in which teachers give information in lectures, the active-learning approach challenges students to reflect, discuss, debate, and problem-solve as primary ways of learning. That is not to say that lectures are out. Nursing students still have to learn facts and information. Some of this information must be memorized. It's just that learning can't stop at memorization. Teachers must use active learning techniques to help students build critical thinking skills.

Chickering and Gamson (1987) reminded us that learning is not a spectator sport. Learning requires that students make what they learn a part of themselves by talking about it and relating it to the world around them. Unfortunately, the desire to memorize is a tough habit to break. Even after starting active learning approaches, Magnussen (2001) noted that some nursing students actually increased their reliance on memorization.

Tips on improving study habits. In terms of time management, first of all, be realistic about what you can accomplish. Nursing school will consume much of your time. You will need to evaluate which activities and responsibilities should be put on the back burner temporarily or, maybe, given up altogether. Some items in your schedule might be easy to toss aside. Other items, such as family responsibilities, may be more difficult to reprioritize. To complicate things further, schedules change from class to class and from semester to semester. The amount of time available to hold down a part-time job may be higher or lower depending upon the semester.

I recommend that you develop a detailed schedule at the beginning of each semester. Record the times your classes are scheduled, the due dates for major assignments, times for lab sessions, and other school requirements. Don't forget to schedule homework and commuting times. Be generous here; don't shortchange yourself on the time it will take to complete your homework. Then, look for open blocks of time in your schedule. It may not seem like much, but you will need to schedule in other high-priority activities. Dunham (2001) suggested that you make the most of your nonschool time by bundling activities. For example, combine errands to save time. Bring one of your kids with you on errands and use that time to catch up on what's happening at your child's school. Listen to taped lectures on your daily commute. Think of other possibilities of how you might cluster your activities.

One common time complaint is the vast amount of required reading. It is not uncommon to have over 100 pages of reading per week on top of other homework. Making efficient use of your reading time becomes important. Ideally, you should read your assigned reading before class. This allows you to understand the lecture or class discussion better. Some students prefer reading the material after class and using their lecture notes to help guide them through the reading. Personally, I am not comfortable with this approach. I find that these students often only read what was talked about in class, and skip over other sections in the assigned reading. This is not wise. Remember, your teacher will not assign reading that is not important. The teacher will not have time enough in class to discuss everything that is given as reading material, but you will still need to know the information. My recommendation is that you complete all the readings, whether before or after class. Use your class notes as a *review* guide, not as a *reading* guide.

Dunham (2001) noted that students must comprehend what they are reading. Time is wasted if you have to reread something over and over again. Dunham suggested reviewing the objectives for each chapter. After reading each section in the book, Dunham recommended asking the following: "What did I just read? What does it mean? Why is it important? How does this apply?" (p. 77). Other tips include highlighting key sections in the reading and taking notes or making an outline as you read. Then, compare those notes later to the notes you took in class. Perhaps the best method presented by Dunham is the SQ3R (Survey-Question-Read-Review-Recite) method, developed by nursing instructor Judy Reishtein. This method recommends that you read the material before class. First start off with surveying the assigned reading. Read the Introduction, review the objectives, end-of-chapter questions, and subheadings in the readings. Second, question yourself as to what the author wants you to learn and what is most important in this material. Third, read the material in a quiet place where you won't be disturbed. Fourth, review the objectives and reread the chapter summary and key sections. And fifth, recite by explaining meanings in the reading and by answering the end-of-chapter questions. Reishtein suggested that you do the first three steps in one night, with the review and recite steps done later in the week.

Dunham (2001) also warned of the problems with procrastination. Many of us put off doing things until later, and student nurses are no different. However, due to the fast pace of nursing school and the large amount of content that must be learned, procrastination can wind up being an express ticket to a class failure. Students who put off working on an assignment until next week find themselves having to finish that assignment on top of new assignments that are now due. These students become more stressed, do not perform their best work, and fall behind. Dunham suggested that students explore why they procrastinate. Some of us find the assignment difficult or boring, so we don't want to finish it. Some of us are fearful that we won't do well. We put off working on the assignment, turn in something at the last minute, and sure enough we earn a poor grade. To overcome this situation, Dunham recommended peer pressure to keep you motivated. Plan with a classmate to have assignments done *early*. Share your work (unless forbidden by your instructor) with your classmate and ask for feedback. Use your classmate's feedback to improve the quality of your work, and have it done on time.

Since time is limited, you must make the most of the time you have allotted for homework. As I mentioned earlier, avoiding distractions while you study will make you more productive. In other words, keeping up on Facebook and watching a favorite movie while you are doing homework will not allow you to concentrate and study. When it is time for homework, find a quiet space and close the door. Turn off your cell phone, and if necessary, post a "Do Not Disturb" sign on the door. Family members or roommates need to understand that when you are doing homework, you are off limits except for an emergency. Better yet, leave the house and go someplace designed for studying, such as the library. Not only does the library have study resources available (such as reference books, computer terminals, etc.), the library allows you to be away from the distractions at home.

Lastly, develop habits that will foster critical thinking. Avoid reading your lecture notes over and over again as you study. This only encourages you to memorize your notes. For difficult material, I tell students to draw the information out on a piece of paper. For example, you could have written in your lecture notes the steps involved of how someone develops pneumonia. Reading the words in your lecture notes only puts the words in your brain's memory banks. Strong connections in the brain don't develop with this limited approach. Instead, get a blank piece of paper and draw out the steps of how someone develops pneumonia. You don't need to be an artist to do this. Stick figures and crude symbols are sufficient. Drawing out the steps forces you to explain to yourself how this process happens. Drawing out the steps also provides a visual image of the process in your memory. After you have drawn out the steps, look back at your notes. Are the steps accurate? Did you leave anything out? Then, to really foster critical thinking, go back to your drawing. Ask yourself questions such as these: "How would things change if this step didn't happen?" "What would happen if the nurse acted here in the drawing....would pneumonia still develop?" "If the person had chronic lung disease, how would this drawing change?" Make changes to your drawing as you answer these questions. These types of drawings are known as concept maps. Concept maps help students more clearly identify concepts and explain how concepts are related to one another. Concept maps help build critical thinking skills (Daley Shaw, Balistrieri, Glassenapp, & Piacentine, 1999; Taylor & Littleton-Kearney, 2011; Wilgis & McConnell, 2008).

Another way to build critical thinking skills is to avoid what I call "flash card study groups," in which students quiz each other with facts, definitions, and information bits. "What is the biggest chamber in the heart?" "What is post-partum depression?" "What is the normal level for blood glucose?" This type of a study group is a waste of your valuable time. First, you can do this type of studying by yourself. Second, this type of study group encourages memorization of information, not critical thinking. Instead, turn your study group into what I call "explanation study groups." These groups only ask questions that require an explanation. "Why is the left ventricle the largest heart chamber?" "How do support groups help women with post-partum depression?" "How does the body respond when the blood glucose drops to 60 mg/dL?" In addition, "what if" questions should be asked as follow-up questions. For example: "What if the left ventricle grows too large?" "What if a woman doesn't have access to a support group?" "What if the body doesn't mount a sufficient response to a low blood glucose level?" This type of questioning forces you to explore nuances, consider different possibilities, and apply your knowledge in different ways. This type of questioning quickly spots areas where your knowledge is weak. Knowing your knowledge gaps helps point you in the right direction for further studying. Most important, this type of questioning is the type of questioning that real nurses use in the clinical setting. Development of critical thinking skills prepares you for the reasoning required to solve clinical practice problems.

Personal and family characteristics and health

Each of us has a different set of personal and family characteristics. Some of these help us be more successful, such as having supportive families who can help out with chores so we have time to study, or provide emotional support and encouragement (Dapremont, 2011; Moceri, 2010). Other characteristics become barriers. For example, Urwin et al. (2010) reviewed a number of studies that reported some students had to leave nursing school because of childcare or other family demands. Childcare and family obligations may be especially challenging for some minority students, due to cultural expectations or lack of access to resources, and for older students (Arnault-Pelletier, Brown, Desjarlais, & McBeth, 2006; Moceri, 2010; Norman, Buerhaus, Donelan, McCloskey, & Dittus, 2005). Others students leave for health reasons. Rouse and Rooda (2010) reported that 5% of the students in their accelerated baccalaureate program left due to their own illness or illness of a family member.

It's easy to understand how these characteristics might be challenging. If you have many family responsibilities or are experiencing illness, you may have much less time for studying or may have to miss class. This increases stress and will decrease your ability to earn good grades. Other characteristics seem less obvious. For example, being the first person in the family to attend college creates a barrier for some students (Childs, Jones, Nugent, & Cook, 2004; Wong, Seago, Keane, & Grumbach, 2008). These families may not understand the demands placed on nursing students, particularly in terms of the amount of time needed for studying. These families may be less willing to relieve students of their responsibilities at home. Also, these families may not have prepared their sons and daughters for college life and culture.

Tips for negotiating family responsibilities

Sometimes, family and friends are unhappy with your school commitments. They want your time, and they feel neglected when you have to leave them to go study. Dunham (2001) stated that nursing students need to sell their program to family and friends. You have to remind them how important nursing school is for you and the family's future. Remind family and friends that your crazy schedule is only temporary. Also, involve family and friends in your studies whenever possible. For example, the kids may be able to help you study for a test by making flash cards for you. Stay in touch with friends by inviting them to join you on campus for a cup of coffee. One student of mine told me that she had her husband develop a computerized schedule for her. Involving others with your school activities helps maintain important personal connections, keeps others informed of your school responsibilities, and helps them feel like they have a part in your important work.

Some family members may forget that your school day doesn't end when you come home. They forget that you have homework that must be completed. Discuss this with your family. Go over your schedule and let them know when you are available and unavailable. For example, "After dinner, I need two hours for homework. After that, I will be available to help out with…." Family members will be more agreeable if they know you will have devoted time to family and home. Also, speak with family members about taking on some of your responsibilities when you aren't available. Sweeten the deal by offering them something special in return. For example, you might say to your spouse, "I know I usually do the dishes every evening. But this week, if you do the dishes so I can do homework, I will treat you to dinner at your favorite restaurant this weekend, plus do the dishes on Saturday and Sunday." Again, remind your family that your school schedule is not permanent. Make plans with your family and friends to spend extra time with them during breaks between semesters.

Some students have caregiving responsibilities at home, such as taking care of small children or an elderly relative. This presents more difficult challenges than reassigning chores or rescheduling relaxation time with family. In these situations, don't be shy about approaching other family members to pitch in and help out. Again, remind them about the importance of school, that your schedule is temporary, and that you'll do something nice for them in return. Don't forget to explore outside resources as well. Some schools offer on-site day care. Speak with your school advisor about resources available on campus. Some communities have social service organizations that provide assistance to caregivers. Explore these organizations and see if you qualify for assistance.

If all else fails, speak with your teachers. If there is a family conflict that cannot be resolved, perhaps your teacher can give you an extension on an assignment. The trick here is to communicate ahead of time with your teachers. Don't just turn in an assignment late without an explanation or explain the lateness after-the-fact. As soon as you become aware of the conflict, talk with your teacher and negotiate some sort of an accommodation. Your teachers understand conflicts with family schedules. Many of them have similar conflicts with their own families. Also, your teachers want you to succeed. Keep your teachers in the loop. Accept any assistance they might offer.

Finances and outside work

Nursing school is expensive. Average annual costs for tuition and room and board in 2009 ranged from $7,567 at public two-year colleges to $31,704 at private four-year universities (U.S. Department of Education, 2010). Again, these are average prices. At my university, full-time nursing students could easily have paid over $46,000 for tuition, room, board, and fees for the 2011–12 school year. On top of this are other expenses, such as the costs of books, additional lab fees, and equipment. Some schools require that you carry health insurance (if you don't already) or malpractice insurance (to protect you if you harm a patient). Of course, there is the cost of a school uniform. Many schools work with local shops to reduce costs, but students often need scrubs, lab coats, special shoes, etc. Some students need to purchase a new computer for school. Most students have the additional costs of paper and printer ink. As you can see, the list can go on and on (Dunham, 2001).

Even at the schools with the cheapest tuition, very few students have enough money to pay for all school expenses out-of-pocket; and few students come to nursing school on full scholarships. This means that most students have to scrimp and save and borrow money to pay all the school expenses. Then, there are the costs of rent, utility bills, and commuting costs for students who live off campus. Financial concerns are some of the leading reasons that students struggle in or leave school (Nursing Standard, 2005; Norman et al., 2005; Urwin et al., 2010). In England, some students were graduating with debts over $36,000 in 2005 and 86% of students had to work while going to school to pay their bills. An American study noted that in 2003, 52% of nursing students used grants and loans as the primary source for paying for their education (Norman et al., 2005). These studies are now out-of-date, but the overall message is the same. At my university, 64% of all undergraduate nursing students had loans to pay for their education in 2011. And prices are only going up. The U.S. Department of Education (2010) noted that college costs rose 32% at public schools between 1998 and 2008. With the increase in costs combined with the recent economic downturn, I can only assume that financial barriers for students will become more worrisome than they have been in the past.

Tips for paying for school

Students have held part-time jobs, sought financial assistance from parents, and applied for grants and scholarships to pay for school. All of these financial resources are still available, but the recent poor economy has made some financial resources harder to come by. With rising unemployment, part-time jobs are harder to find. Financial help from parents may be scarce if one or both are unemployed. Foundations and health care organizations are more limited in their ability to provide scholarships and grants. Worse yet, as the government trims costs and programs in order to address the federal budget deficit, the long-term availability of government-supported grants and student loans is unclear. These new realities are likely to cause higher levels of stress than I experienced as a student.

Today, students often must piece together small amounts of money from many different sources to pay for school. It often takes a lot of detective work to find enough money sources that can be pooled together to build a financial package that is going to work. A good place to start your financial search is the student aid website at the U.S. Department of Education (http://www.studentaid.ed.gov). Although not specific to nursing students, this website has general information about the types of financial aid available and the Free Application for Federal Student Aid (FAFSA) form. The FAFSA must be completed by all students requesting government-supported financial aid. Second, contact the financial aid office at the schools you hope to attend. These offices will guide you through the application process and how to assemble a financial aid package. Many schools offer scholarships and other types of assistance to qualified students. These offices will have information on these opportunities. If you already work for a health care organization, speak with your human resources office. Many companies offer some assistance to employees who want to further their education. And of course, be sure to explore private sources of money. Some banks offer student loans. Some foundations still offer scholarships for nursing students, especially for minority students or students who meet various eligibility requirements. An Internet search will pull up options for you to explore (Dunham, 2001; Pelican News, 2007).

Some students are reluctant to apply for student loans. Some students are worried about graduating with a large debt that must be paid back, particularly in these economic times when nursing jobs may take longer to find after graduation than they did in the past. In order to avoid loans, some students take on full-time jobs to pay for school. Too often, however, these working students find that they don't have time to study, sleep, or both. This situation puts students in danger of failing their classes, or at least, not producing their best work. These students may shortchange themselves of a quality education, or an education altogether (Drill, 2010).

I recommend that you don't reject loans outright. Sure, you should limit your debt. Too many of us let our bills pile up beyond our ability to pay for them. But student loans should be viewed as an investment in your future. Student loans are not all that different than loans to purchase a home. Few people have enough money to buy a house with cash. Most home buyers take out a loan. A wise home purchase is a good investment. Student loans can be a wise investment too. A student loan may be the only way to free yourself from having to work full-time while you are going to school. However, your student loan package must be a wise one. First, borrow as little as possible. Get as much money as you can from scholarships, savings, grants, and a job with reasonable hours before figuring out how much money to borrow. Second, get loans with the lowest interest rates possible. Generally, government loans have much lower interest rates than do loans from banks. Third, make sure you are clear about the repayment schedule and the terms of the loan. Different lenders have different requirements. Some lenders make you start repaying your loan right after you finish school; others allow a grace period, which gives you enough time to find a good job before you have to start making payments. Some lenders allow you to pay off the loan over many years; others make you repay your loan in a relatively short time. The bottom line is this: in these uncertain economic times, *all* financing options must be considered—and considered carefully.

Once you get financial aid, make sure you understand the requirements for keeping the aid you will receive. For most types of financial aid, you must stay in school, often full-time. Most sources require that students earn passing grades or higher, but there may be other less-than-obvious requirements too. For example, many students do not know that illegal behavior, even misdemeanors, can result in losing your financial aid (Alcohol & Drug Abuse Weekly, 2006). According to the U.S. Department of Education (2011), students can lose their financial aid if they are convicted for selling or possessing illegal drugs. Certain types of sexual offences may also result in the loss of financial aid. In many nursing schools, these types of crimes will result in expulsion from the school. Students may be able to transfer to another nursing school, or change majors, but they will have to do so without financial aid. These students may find college too expensive and drop out of school completely. In short, financial aid requires that you stay in school, earn good grades, and *stay out of trouble*.

Coping styles

Barriers cause high levels of stress, which leads to anxiety (Deary et al., 2003; Timmons & Kaliszer, 2002). The high levels of stress and anxiety among nursing students have been topics of much research since the 1970s (Watson et al., 2008). Many of these studies have examined the causes of stress, and the increased stress that happens when multiple barriers are combined. Some authors suggested that schools could provide students with stress-reducing resources such as tutoring, mentorship, and meditation and relaxation (Moscaritolo, 2009). The obvious thinking here is that students will be more successful if their stress levels are reduced. However, other authors examined stress by studying the personality traits and coping skills of nursing students. Deary et al. (2003) reported that some personality traits are shaped by genetics and upbringing. Some people are naturally more anxious and do not handle stress well. These traits are difficult to change. After following a group of nursing students through their entire school program, these researchers noted that naturally anxious students displayed more worry and insecurity as time went on. Students who were more irritable, more selfish, and less conscientious were more likely to leave school than other students. On the other hand, being conscientious is a positive trait and strongly predicts success for male nursing students in Taiwan (Lou et al., 2010). Although we don't know enough about the complex relationships among personality, stress, and success in school to warrant personality tests for students applying to nursing school, Deary et al. suggested that schools identify negative traits early in a student's career. Early identification of negative traits will allow teachers to reach out to students earlier, hopefully before problems start to occur.

Deary et al. (2003) also looked at the coping abilities of nursing students. Coping is a broad term that describes efforts people make to address stress-related problems (Lazarus & Folkman, 1984). Much has been written about different types of coping and which ways of coping seem to work the best. Deary et al. reported that coping ability, like personality, is generally stable. People develop their preferred style of coping, and then use that style in most situations that they find stressful. Figuring out your coping style can help you understand yourself better. It also helps you learn how to change your coping style when necessary, which, in turn, improves your ability to cope with stress.

Coping styles can be labeled as task-oriented, emotion-oriented, or avoidance-oriented (Deary et al., 2003). In task-oriented coping (problem-focused coping), people correctly identify the issues and set goals to address those issues. People using this style seek information and help when needed. In many situations, task-oriented coping leads to more immediate and direct problem-solving. It promotes creativity and self-sufficiency. In emotion-oriented coping, people focus on their feelings about the challenges they encounter. They try to reframe or minimize the problem, blame themselves or others, or suppress problems (Boyd, 2002). In avoidance-oriented coping, people avoid issues with distractions. This helps them get their minds off their problems (Deary et al., 2003). Distractions can include recreation activities or spending time with friends. Sometimes, these distractions can be harmful such as using alcohol to forget one's problems.

It would appear that task-oriented coping is superior above the other coping styles, but this assumption is premature. Not all situations are appropriate for task-oriented coping. Sometimes, emotion-oriented or avoidance-oriented actions are helpful. For example, let's say you are on your way to school. You leave the house in plenty of time, but there is an accident on the freeway. Now you are stuck in traffic. You will be late for school. You find yourself growing anxious. You fear your teacher will scold you for being late. In this situation, there is nothing you can do to solve the immediate problem. You cannot make the cars move any faster. Instead, you can use emotion-oriented coping to reframe the problem and reflect on your response to the problem. Your late arrival to class is not due to your own poor time management, but rather, due to the unpredictable nature of our world. There was nothing you could have done to prevent this problem. Therefore, there is no need for guilt or for self-criticism. As the traffic snarl continues, you are feeling more anxious about being late. Ask yourself, "How will my anxiousness help this situation?" The answer, obviously, is that it won't help. You now focus on reducing your anxiety by using distraction. You practice deep breathing exercises and turn on some soft music. You accept the fact that you will arrive to class late; you won't let this fact ruin your day. You tell yourself, "it is what it is" (one of my favorite sayings). Remember, the purpose of coping is to reduce stress, not always to reverse or solve the problem that is causing the stress.

The point here is this: there are multiple coping styles. Each of us has a preferred style, and some styles work better in some situations than in others. To cope most effectively, each of us must become skilled at using all types of styles. If you use only task-oriented coping, you will feel like you have lost control and become quite angry and anxious in situations for which you have very little control. In the traffic example above, the task-oriented person could develop road rage. If you use only emotion-focused coping, you may not explore the causes of problems or their solutions. Instead you may focus too much on how you feel about your problems, which could lead to a sense that you are always a victim of things going on around you. If you use only avoidance-oriented coping, you run the risk of ignoring problems altogether. Problems that don't receive your attention will only grow larger and create new problems. Others will see you as immature, or worse, wonder if you have lost touch with reality. Each coping style has some good, but if taken to the extreme, each coping style can lead to problems, which reminds me of my other favorite saying: too much of a good thing is always a bad thing!

Tips on coping with stress

In addition to exploring your preferred coping style, you need to find multiple ways to manage your stress. There are an unlimited number of things you can do to relieve stress, so a good place to start is to use stress-relieving activities that have worked for you in the past. Your familiarity with these activities will make it easier for you to use them when the stress from school starts to build. However, some of your favorite activities may not be appropriate. For example, let's assume your favorite stress reliever is to spend a weekend fishing with friends. But now that you are in school and your schedule is tight, you may not be able to get away for a whole weekend. Now what? You will need to find other activities that you can do in less amount of time, or even by yourself, that will give you about the same level of stress relief. This will take some exploration and some trial and error, but you will need to find different ways to relieve your stress. You will need to find stress-relieving methods that you can use on the spur of a moment (such as deep breathing exercises when you find out there will be a pop quiz in class), as well as methods that you can plan into your schedule.

This last point, planning methods into your schedule, is very important. Many of us forget to put rest and relaxation times into our already overflowing schedules. When we become busy, we often get rid of rest and relaxation time because we see this time as something that is optional. Sayles and Shelton (2005) reported that forgetting to schedule rest and relaxation will make you a worn-out learner. If you are worn-out, you won't be successful. They offered a model for rest and relaxation that I really like. The model includes two pieces: FRED and PAL. FRED stands for Fun-Rest-Exercise-Diet. Each of us must schedule times for fun activities, times for rest (sleep-deprived students quickly become poor students), times for exercise, and enough time to eat a healthy diet (eating on the run often leads to poor nutrition). PAL stands for Praise-Advise-Listen and speaks to the emotional component of stress reduction. They recommended that we praise ourselves and others. This will boost morale and confidence. Also, we must accept the advice and help that is offered to us. This means that we must listen. "Just listen; you never know what you may learn" (p. 100). By using FRED and PAL, you will maintain the physical and emotional stamina to cope with the stress of being a nursing student and employ reasonable distraction activities that will make stress reduction fun.

Barriers Caused by School Factors

Some barriers are created by factors that shape the culture and the policies of the nursing school. These factors by themselves may not cause problems for some students, but when combined with some of the individual factors just discussed, the total level of barriers can rise to a point that some students cannot overcome.

Schedules

Earlier, I discussed time management. Students must become experts at juggling multiple commitments from school, work, family, and self. On top of this, students have to work around the academic schedules that are set by the school. These schedules can create significant barriers for students who have limited wiggle room in their personal schedules. Many students find academic schedules to be rigid. Some students get angry because they believe that teachers do not care that the schedules create problems. But schedules have to be set, and no matter the schedule, *someone* will be unhappy. For example, maybe your pharmacology class is scheduled for Tuesday and Thursday mornings. These mornings conflict with your late-night work schedule. You would prefer that the class was held on Tuesday and Thursday evenings. But evenings may not work for others in the class who have childcare responsibilities, or for the teacher who would like to spend time with his or her family in the evenings. Other days and times may not work either because the classrooms are booked for other classes. You can easily see the limits.

Clinical schedules can be even more rigid. Students are scheduled when the clinical site can accommodate students. Schools have little control over the schedules set by hospitals and clinics. To make matters worse, schedules can change every semester or term. Your clinical one semester may be scheduled for Tuesday and Wednesday mornings; but the next semester, your clinical is scheduled for Thursday and Friday evenings. These changing schedules create chaos for students as they negotiate the changes with family, friends, and employers. Keeping yourself and others informed about your changing schedule as soon as those changes are known will help reduce planning problems. Otherwise, there is little you can do to prevent the changes from happening. Ask family members and employers to be as flexible as they can with your schedule changes.

Incivility

Incivility has become the new buzzword in nursing education. Incivility can be loosely defined as rude, inappropriate, disrespectful, and unprofessional behaviors that create a difficult or hostile environment. Incivility can include behaviors that are mildly annoying and insulting all the way up to violent outbursts (Clark & Springer, 2007; Luparell, 2007). Perhaps the most extreme cases of incivility occurred in 2002 when a nursing student shot and killed three nursing professors in Arizona, and again in 2012 when classmates were shot at a California nursing school. Several authors have reviewed articles on incivility and have reported that most articles discussed students' uncivil behavior toward their teachers (Suplee, Lachman, Siebert, & Anselmi, 2008; Luparell, 2011; Marchiondo, Marchiondo, & Lasiter, 2010). Student incivility includes behaviors such as sarcastic remarks, inappropriate cell phone use in class, cheating, having side conversations in class or ignoring the teacher, coming to class late or skipping class, demanding special favors from teachers, and confronting and threatening teachers in anger. Luparell (2004) noted that most cases of incivility arose when teachers gave students negative criticism on their performance or when students earned failing grades.

Marchiondo et al. (2010) reported that some authors believed that student incivility is on the rise. There are some thoughts to explain this rise. Some believed that today's nursing students are less prepared emotionally and academically for the demands of nursing school; others noted generational differences in etiquette and values; others noted a general increase in rudeness in society due to selfishness; and others noted that strong interpersonal communication skills have decreased since technology has allowed people to communicate without talking to each other face-to-face (Suplee et al., 2008; Marchiondo et al., 2010). This last point has received a lot of attention. I agree that emails, text messaging, and tweets have changed communication etiquette for the worse. Polite and professional communication takes practice. Students who frequently use electronics to communicate don't get this practice. These students come to nursing school with poorer communication skills than did students a generation ago.

Regardless of the causes, student incivility is very damaging to the learning environment. Luparell (2007) reported that student incivility takes a physical and emotional toll on teachers. Teachers spend more time with uncivil students by trying to address the students' concerns, monitoring their behavior, or disciplining these students. Ultimately, teachers experience more stress, poor sleep, more anxiety, and dissatisfaction with their jobs. Student incivility can erode the self-esteem of faculty and even lead to posttraumatic stress disorder (a disorder commonly seen in soldiers and rape victims). Some teachers have cited student incivility as a primary reason for quitting their jobs. In response, some teachers may give in to an uncivil student's demands simply to avoid a fight. Teachers have reported changing their assignments just to make students happy. I have seen this personally. I remember one professor telling me that it is just easier to give students what they want than to risk conflict with students. Other teachers give higher grades to students than were deserved out of fear of being criticized or facing possible legal action (Boley & Whitney, 2003; Luhanga, Yonge, & Myrick, 2008). Obviously, this response doesn't foster learning and only rewards the student for bad behavior.

I recently experienced a very difficult uncivil student. This student started disrupting my class by talking to her neighbors and texting on her cell phone. I asked her to see me after class. I explained how her behavior was disrupting to me and to other students. She agreed to stop, but the behavior continued every time I turned my back. When I would catch her being disruptive, I would stop my lecture and simply look at her until she quieted down. This usually provoked an angry stare from her. After the first exam, the student demanded that I meet with her and explain why I gave her such a poor grade. (I reminded her that grades were not something I gave, but rather, grades were something that students earned.) Later in my office, I went over her exam with her. I asked her questions and listened to her explanations. It was clear to me that she had not studied for the test. She continued to do poorly in the class. I met with her again to offer suggestions on study habits and how to prepare for the exams. At our second meeting, she made it clear to me that she didn't like the class, didn't think the material I was teaching was important, and that she didn't have time to study. She ignored my suggestions and shared with the other students that I was an awful teacher. Ultimately, she failed the course. She was very angry and told me that she was going to fight my unfair grade. Soon, I heard that her parents were meeting with the associate dean to discuss the student's grade. One of my coworkers asked me if I knew who the student was. "Of course," I replied. "I've worked with this student all semester." What I didn't know was that the student came from a wealthy family who had given millions to the university. Some wondered if I should change the grade. If I angered her parents, the university might suffer. But I stood my ground. I could not in good conscience say that she passed the class when she did not.

I was not invited to the meeting. This bothered me greatly because I could not defend my actions. I assumed that her parents would be like some parents I had met in the past. These parents could not believe that their child was anything but exceptional. They could not believe that their child skipped class, didn't show interest or motivation, or was disrespectful. They assumed that the teacher was either unfair to their child, was incompetent, or both. Fortunately, the associate dean reviewed all the evidence with the student's parents. After a lengthy meeting, her parents realized that their daughter did not earn a passing grade. The student was forced to repeat the class.

This experience could have been very demoralizing for me. It came only a few months after the parents of a different student swooped on campus with a lawyer to fight the grade I gave their son. I was not invited to that meeting either. In both situations, my integrity was challenged. In effect, I felt as if I was on trial without being allowed to sit in the courtroom. Both situations ended in my favor due largely to supportive administrators at my university. Regardless, my nerves were rattled. After these experiences, I understood how some teachers might give students better marks just to avoid these kinds of battles.

Teachers aren't the only victims of student incivility. Student incivility hurts the student as well. If students use uncivil actions to get what they want, students are not likely to get what they need to get a quality education. Students may graduate thinking they have the knowledge required for good nursing practice when, in reality, they do not. Also, students do not develop the values and ethics required of nurses, particularly the values of respect, professionalism, and nonjudgmental attitudes (Luparell, 2011). Suplee et al. (2008) commented on a common uncivil student behavior: excessive defensiveness to criticism. They stated

> Excessive defensiveness can prevent students from learning from their mistakes. Recognizing and avoiding excessive defensiveness is not easy if the student has developed a pattern of protecting a fragile self-esteem in this way. Individuals with a healthy self-esteem are able to admit their mistakes. Giving constructive feedback on student performance is part of every professor's job. But not all students understand that their role is to at least listen and examine the feedback for the truth. (p. 72)

Most important, uncivil students who do not change their behaviors can graduate and become uncivil nurses. These nurses often become bullies in the workplace. These nurses threaten healthy relationships with coworkers and with patients. These nurses put themselves at risk for being fired.

On the other hand, teachers can also display uncivil behaviors toward students. Marchiondo et al. (2010) said that the effects of teacher incivility have not been given enough attention by researchers, due to unawareness, embarrassment, and denial of the problem. They stated that the problem needs attention because teacher incivility creates a culture that sparks student incivility, a negative tit-for-tat. Uncivil teacher behaviors include coming to class late, changing assignments without notice, unfair grading practices, inflexibility, ignoring disruptive student behaviors, giving confusing and wandering lectures, berating students in public, belittling or taunting students, using threats, singling out students for punishment, as well as other disrespectful actions (Clark & Springer, 2007; Marchiondo et al.). Most important, teacher incivility creates a negative environment that hampers student creativity and learning. These authors found that most students either talked with each other about teacher incivility or just put up with it. One third of the students they studied cried and felt anxious or depressed about the uncivil behavior. Less than 20% of the students ever reported the problem to the teacher or to school officials.

Marchiondo et al. (2011) outlined four major consequences of teacher incivility. First, incivility raises student stress and anxiety in nursing programs that are already very stressful. Incivility can stretch students' abilities to cope with the demands placed on them, leading students to feel hopeless and desperate. Second, teacher incivility can lower the safety of students' clinical performance. Students find themselves in complex situations in the clinical setting. They need to trust teachers and feel comfortable in asking questions in order to provide safe care to patients. Third, nursing is a caring profession. Uncivil teachers violate the ethics of care. They provide a negative role model for students. And fourth, teacher incivility decreases the satisfaction and trust students have in their schools.

Tips on facing incivility

Incivility only survives in an environment of silence. People stay silent for many reasons including embarrassment, fear, and uncertainty. People may recognize incivility and may feel uncomfortable with incivility, but when they stay silent, the person causing the incivility gets the message that his or her behavior is acceptable. With silence, the uncivil person is not made aware of the behavior, which only encourages the behavior to continue. Therefore, the best way to combat incivility is to speak up. I know that this is often easier said than done.

Speaking up may be particularly difficult if you need to tell your teacher that he or she is uncivil. For these types of difficult conversations, you might find the *Crucial Conversations* method helpful (Patterson, Grenny, McMillan, & Switzler, 2012). This method challenges each of us to reflect before we speak up. This reflection is designed to help us clarify the message that needs to be delivered. The method then guides us to stay in control of the message, speak persuasively and not abrasively, and stay open to hearing the comments of others. Regardless of whether you use this method or another to guide you through a tense conversation, the conversation needs to occur. Patterson et al. (2012) noted that when we stay silent, the increased stress and anger can lead to violence. This violence may be displayed as gossip, nasty written comments on students' evaluations of the teacher, or even by verbal and physical assaults. In order to prepare for this conversation, you might find the assistance of a school advisor or mentor helpful.

In addition to speaking up, I recommend that you participate in student groups to establish clearly written policies that define uncivil behaviors and describe procedures for addressing incivility. Many schools have these policies in place, but some policies may need revisions or expansion. Suplee et al. (2008) provided excellent topics that should be included in incivility policies. Ask your school to make incivility a topic for seminars, teacher development sessions, and student orientation sessions. Work with teachers to establish ground rules for the classroom. Good examples of some ground rules include not interrupting presenters, not wording questions with sarcasm, and keeping online postings respectful and constructive (Suplee et al. 2008). Most important, become a role model to others for civil and professional behaviors.

Progression policies

Most students understand that poor grades can prevent success. Unlike some majors, a failing grade in a nursing class usually prevents a student from moving forward. These students must repeat failed courses, which can delay their graduation date by as much as 12 months. However, many students are surprised to learn that nursing schools have other requirements about whether or not students can move forward in the program. These requirements are called progression policies. For example, many schools have a limit as to how many times a student can repeat a course. At my school, students can repeat a required course only once. Also, students cannot fail more than one nursing course. Contrary to what some of our students think, this policy is not designed to weed out poor students. All students in our school are bright and capable; otherwise, they would not have been admitted into the nursing program. Instead, students who fail more than one course are usually experiencing one or more of the barriers already discussed. Perhaps their family and work schedules don't allow them enough time for homework. Perhaps their study habits need improvement. Perhaps they don't cope well with stress. These students often need to take some time away from school to work on their challenges. Then they can return to nursing school in a better position for success.

Other progression policies are becoming more common. For example, many schools require that students pass a standardized exam in order to move forward. (Standardized nursing exams are tests that are given to a large national group of nursing students. The exam uses the same group of questions and scoring method for each student. These exams allow for comparison among students from different schools.) Spurlock (2006) reported that schools use these types of policies to improve their students' success on the National Council Licensure Examination for Registered Nurses (NCLEX-RN®) exam, the exam you must pass to earn your nursing license. State boards of nursing monitor how well students from each school perform on this exam as a way to mark a school's quality. If a school's graduates do poorly on this exam for several years in a row, that school may come under review by the state, may be forced to make sweeping changes, or even be closed due to poor quality. In order to boost pass rates on the NCLEX-RN, many schools make students take standardized exams that are designed to predict whether or not a student will pass the NCLEX-RN. If a student does not pass standardized exams, he or she may have to review material and retake the exam. If a student still cannot pass a standardized exam, the school may prevent the student from taking the NCLEX-RN exam without further action.

Spurlock (2006) criticized these policies as being too harsh. He said that using a standardized exam as a requirement for a diploma is high-stakes testing, a practice that has been denounced by education experts. High-stakes testing creates an excessive level of anxiety for students and may not truly reflect a student's level of knowledge. Commercially prepared exams claim to predict which students will be successful on the NCLEX-RN exam, but Spurlock noted that many other factors influence success on the NCLEX-RN. (These factors are discussed in Chapter 7.) According to Spurlock, what these tests should do is predict which students will *fail* the NCLEX-RN. If these tests could do that, then teachers could identify these students and provide them with appropriate supports and resources to help them improve. Also, standardized exams have been criticized for showing racial bias by using language and requiring students to think in ways that are not always the same as those used by racial minorities or by those whose primary language is not English. Finally, Spurlock said that using only one test score for a decision to allow a student to take the NCLEX-RN exam is downright unethical and goes against the values of the nursing profession.

Although Spurlock's warnings are important to consider, I believe his criticisms are overly dramatic. Most of the nursing schools with which I am familiar do not use only one test score for progression decisions. Most schools use many different types of data to make progression decisions. For example, in addition to grades, many schools use student performance and behavior in the lab or clinical setting as a progression requirement. Some schools consider a student's writing and speaking ability as a factor for progression. Also, many schools use a series of learning modules and smaller standardized exams to evaluate students instead of the score on one big standardized exam at the end of their program. These smaller exams help teachers and students see which areas need improvement as they occur during the program. Some schools have clearly written guidelines on how to help students improve before they move forward in the program. Other schools use portfolios in addition to the exams to document student performance and student readiness for taking the NCLEX-RN exam.

Regardless, more and more schools are adding standardized exams to help determine whether or not students are qualified to take the NCLEX-RN exam. In August 2011, a publisher of nursing standardized exams claimed that over 2,000 nursing schools nationwide used their standardized exams (Assessment Technologies Institute, 2011). Using these exams may actually be helpful to students. Since 2008, the number of students who passed the NCLEX-RN exam on their first try has been higher than it was in the years between 2000 and 2005. By the middle of 2011, over 90% of students passed the exam on the first try—something that hasn't happened since 1995 (National Council of State Boards of Nursing, 2011). It's possible that making sure that students are ready to take the NCLEX-RN exam *before* they take the exam is improving success.

Spurlock (2006) recommended that schools use other strategies to measure student achievement. One strategy he offered was requiring teachers to adopt stronger standards for issuing grades. If grades truly reflected student achievement, then standardized testing would not be necessary. I agree with Spurlock on this point, but making teachers issue grades that students honestly deserve is difficult. Grade inflation, the practice of giving better grades than what was earned or having low requirements for high grades, is too common in nursing education (Boley & Whitney, 2003; Luhanga et al., 2008). Reasons for grade inflation in nursing classes include student incivility and student threats, lack of training on how to evaluate students, lack of clear evaluation guidelines, and a desire to spare students stress (Luhanga et al., 2008). I recently experienced a serious case of grade inflation. One of my poorest students was assigned a clinical experience in an intensive care unit.

His clinical teacher gave him perfect scores in all categories because the student was "nice, pleasant to work with, and eager to learn." Although it is wonderful to have nice students who are eager to learn, students must also gain knowledge and demonstrate that they can safely solve complex patient problems. His teacher did not evaluate knowledge or whether or not he could provide nursing care safely. Grade inflation benefits no one, especially the future patients of unprepared students. Patients want their nurses to be competent, not just nice. Until teachers have the will, freedom, and support to issue grades that students truly earn, standardized exams will be necessary to document student knowledge objectively.

Tips on how to do well on standardized exams

The most important tip for success on a standardized exam is to be prepared for the exam as best as possible. Obviously, you need to study and review the information that will be covered on the exam. Earlier in this chapter, I reviewed how to improve your study habits. Beyond this, there are other ways to prepare for standardized exams. Dunham (2001) suggested that you learn as much as you can about the exam. Read any information and instructions your teacher gives you about the exam. Often, there are practice questions and exams available. Review these questions and take any practice exams that might be offered. This will give you a good sense as to how the questions are worded and the pace of the exam. Also, practice exams will usually let you know what topics you need to study further. These topics should take priority in your study time as you prepare for the exam.

Speaking of time, it is usually better to study for these exams in multiple short sessions instead of cramming for an exam a few days before the exam is scheduled. At my school, students are required to take nine standardized exams. The exams are usually given near the end of each semester. Students have all semester to study and review for an exam, but too many students wait until the very end to open the review books and work on the practice questions. This approach does not allow your brain the time it needs to make strong connections with the material. Information isn't used to build your knowledge; instead, information is crammed into memory banks that may already be overflowing. Not surprisingly, students using this approach usually don't do well on standardized exams. Some teachers make assignments to force students to review and learn material for standardized exams while they are learning the material for the class. This may be helpful, but the responsibility to be prepared for the exam is yours.

On the day of the exam, your brain and your body need to be well rested and ready to go. Busy schedules combined with poor time management makes many nursing students not get enough sleep by staying up late studying the night before an exam. The research on brain function and lack of sleep is quite clear: sleep deprivation reduces many types of brain functioning, including your ability to learn and remember (Chee & Chuah, 2008; Halbach, Spann, & Egan, 2003). My suggestion to you is this: study in the days before the standardized exam. The night before the exam, go to bed early and get plenty of rest. Do not get up extra early to study. This only shortens the amount of time you sleep. Instead, get up only after adequate sleep. When you do get up, do some light exercise (to get your blood pumping), eat a nutritious meal (to feed your brain and body), and build your confidence by telling yourself positive messages. If you must review the material, only skim it the morning of the exam.

You will also need to keep your anxiety down and stay focused. Dunham (2001) suggested taking a few minutes for deep breathing just before the exam. During the exam, if you feel anxious, close your eyes and take a few deep breaths. This will only take a few seconds, but can do much to lower your anxiety. There are many places to look for test-taking tips. My recent Google search turned up at least 20 sites for students. Many of these sites give much of the same information: pace yourself during the exam, read the questions carefully and thoroughly, mark your answers clearly, answer the easier questions first, and ask the teacher for clarification (if that is allowed). Many standardized exams have multiple-choice questions. The websites I reviewed recommended that you read the question before looking at the possible answers, eliminate the answers you know are wrong, read *all* the choices before answering the question, and don't be overly afraid to change answers (but only if you know that your answer is wrong—often your first answer is correct). In my experience, different students seem to have different problems. Some students assume they know the answer to a question before they have even finished reading the question. This often leads to a wrong answer. Other students spend too much time on hard questions and don't finish the test. Still others get too anxious during the test and can't think straight. I suggest that you meet with your teachers or with a counselor at your school's learning center to explore any test-taking weaknesses. Then, use the resources available to you at your school and on-line for tips tailored for your weaknesses.

One last thing: standardized exams, including the NCLEX-RN exam, are now using computerized adaptive testing (CAT) methods. CAT uses computer technology to give students questions that aren't too hard or too easy. Each time you answer a question, the computer calculates your ability. Your next question is leveled so that you have a 50–50 chance of getting it right. If you are answering questions correctly, the test gets harder; if you are answering questions incorrectly, the test gets easier. After a number of questions, the computer is able to accurately predict your ability and decide if your ability level is passing or failing for that exam (National Council of State Boards of Nursing, 2012). It can be upsetting the first time you take an exam with CAT, especially if you are used to earning high grades on exams. If you know the material and are a good test-taker, you usually find many of the questions fairly easy. You finish the exam feeling confident that you did well. This is not always the case in the exam with CAT. Even excellent students miss lots of questions because the computer keeps giving them harder questions. Excellent students leave these exams wondering if they failed. Just remember, it's the *specific* questions that are answered right or wrong that determines your success or failure on this type of an exam, not how *many* questions are answered right. I will talk more about the NCLEX-RN exam in Chapter 7.

Quality of teachers

In the past, most nursing instructors never had formal education on how to teach (Wittmann-Price & Godshall, 2009). They were simply expert nurses who everyone assumed would be expert teachers. Teachers often taught by repeating the habits of their own teachers (good and bad) and by trial-and-error. My own journey as a teacher is typical. I developed expertise as a nurse. At the hospital, I trained new employees and worked with nursing students. I enjoyed teaching, so took on part-time work as a clinical teacher for a local nursing school. I received no instruction on how to teach; I was simply told who to call if I had questions. I quickly learned that teaching nursing students was very different than training new employees. I wasn't given any feedback on my teaching. Since the students seemed to be happy, I assumed that I was a good teacher. After a couple of years, I decided to become a full-time teacher, both in the classroom and in the clinical setting. I took a job at a university-based nursing program. This time, I did receive more information, but most of the information focused on how to work at the university (e.g., how to order books, how to request media equipment). Not much information was given to me on how to teach. I soon found ways to learn more about teaching. I went to conferences, read articles, took some college courses, and sought out the guidance of mentors. It took me several years, but I finally learned some basic principles about teaching. I'm still learning. Each year I learn something new about how to be a better teacher.

Few nursing students in graduate school learn how to be good teachers. Although more schools are now offering classes on teaching, not enough students take these classes. In Chapter 4, Boatright discussed the teacher shortage. According to the AACN (2011), over 67,000 qualified students applying to nursing school were turned away in 2010, mostly because schools didn't have enough teachers. To try to meet the demand, schools are scrambling to attract expert nurses to take jobs as teachers. Some of these new teachers may not be well-prepared to teach students.

McDonald (2010) reviewed the research and reported that nurses who take on teaching jobs face a challenging role transition. First, there is a knowledge curve. New teachers have to learn about new responsibilities and expectations, how to develop lectures and learning activities, how to grade students accurately, how to use new computer programs and other technologies, and everything else that teachers must know. Second, new teachers find themselves in a different environment. The school setting is very different from the clinical setting. Schools have unique cultures, norms, and support systems. Third, new teachers often have to accept lower wages and increased workload than advanced clinical nurses. McDonald estimated that she worked over 50 hours per week during her first year as a teacher. My experience was similar. For a new teacher, this transition can be extremely stressful, especially if the school does not provide enough training and support for new teachers. Poorly prepared teachers are an obvious concern for students. These teachers are not likely to provide quality teaching, which is vital to quality learning.

Fortunately, much information is available in books and articles that can help teachers become better teachers. This information is well-researched and written by education experts. For example, Rossetti and Fox (2009) interviewed 35 college teachers who had won the Presidential Teaching Award at a university in Illinois. These expert teachers had four characteristics. First, expert teachers are present for their students both in body and in mind. Expert teachers build relationships with their students, gain their trust, and keep the students' needs in mind. Second, they promote quality learning. Expert teachers have high standards and hold students to high expectations. These teachers work tirelessly to encourage, support, and mentor their students to meet these expectations. Third, expert teachers are learners themselves. They seek out new knowledge and new ways of doing things. They are not stagnant and outdated. And fourth, expert teachers are enthusiastic. They show their passion for teaching, spark interest, and applaud student success.

In 2005, the National League for Nursing (NLN) launched a new program to recognize expert nursing teachers (Wittman-Price & Godshall, 2009). Building on research on what makes an excellent teacher, the NLN developed an examination process in which teachers could demonstrate their expertise in teaching and become certified as expert teachers. This exam evaluates teachers on their knowledge of how to foster learning, foster student development, encourage good academic behaviors among students, use of expert knowledge to evaluate students, and other teaching skills. Teachers must also demonstrate that they strive to become better teachers. This teacher examination process is setting new ground for helping expert nurses become expert teachers. By 2010, nearly 2,000 nurse educators were certified (National League of Nursing, 2011b). The number of certified teachers grows each year.

Tips for improving the quality of teachers

Too often, students don't recognize that their teachers are learners too. Just as students want and need helpful and constructive feedback on their work, teachers want and need the same. Most schools provide students an opportunity to give teachers feedback. Often this feedback is anonymous so that students will feel free to be honest. Unfortunately, too many students use the anonymous feedback form to complain, air grievances, or write personal attacks against their teachers. These kinds of comments do nothing to improve the quality of teaching. Instead, they confuse and demoralize the teachers. Some comments my coworkers and I have received are nothing more than outright verbal assaults.

To really be helpful, give meaningful feedback to your teachers. Let them know what they did well in supporting your learning. Let them know where they fell short, but don't resort to personal attacks or abrasive language. Let them know what you found difficult with the class, but also let them know if you thought any of the assignments were too easy. Most important, be specific. Vague comments, such as the class was too hard, do not give enough information to be useful. Here's an example of a well-written evaluation for a teacher I will call Mrs. Johnson.

Mrs. Johnson shows great enthusiasm for the students. Each class, she points out the areas we are doing well on in our homework. If there are areas that aren't so good, she provides us additional resources to help us learn and invites us to meet with her to review any material we have questions about. Her lectures are well-organized and easy to follow. She takes time in class to give examples of how the information might be applied in the clinical setting. However, I found the first few lectures and the first exam to be too easy. Mrs. Johnson reviewed material we had already learned. She did not challenge us to apply this information in new ways. I did not feel challenged until we got to the book chapters several weeks into the course. I would recommend that she review this material more quickly and spend more time on the more difficult topics in the course.

From this evaluation, Mrs. Johnson knows to continue applauding the students for their accomplishments, to continue to provide resources, and offer her assistance through student meetings. Mrs. Johnson also learns that she should revise the first portion of the course so that students are building new knowledge onto what they have already learned. This evaluation is meaningful and constructive.

Barriers Caused by Social/Economic Factors

The last category of factors described by Urwin et al. (2010) is one that stems from political and professional sources. However, Urwin et al. come from the United Kingdom, a nation with a nationalized health care system. Some of the factors they discussed, such as low government wages for nurses, don't apply well to American nurses. In a broader look at this category, most of the factors these authors described pertain to issues in the larger society and the current economic picture. Therefore, I have renamed this category as "Social/Economic Factors." This category includes the smallest number of factors, but these factors can create significant barriers nonetheless.

One potential barrier, a negative image of nursing, has received much attention. For example, Gordon (2005) described how the media, especially movies and television programs, show nurses in a very negative light. Clearly, a negative image could persuade some people that nursing is a poor career choice. Family and friends might discourage promising students from applying to nursing school. The number of students entering the field could drop, and some current nurses might leave nursing as they are lured away to more attractive careers. However, a study by Donelan, Buerhaus, DesRoches, Dittus, and Dutwin (2008) rejected the idea of a media that is harmful to nursing. In their national survey, they reported that the first things that come to mind when the general public was asked about nurses were words like "knowledgeable, caring, hardworking, skilled" and other positive images. Also, in a comparison to other professions, they found that only teachers had more respect from the public than did nurses. One in four people reported that they considered becoming nurses, but didn't because of time conflicts or difficult education requirements. All this in spite of the fact that 60% of the public watched shows and movies that had nurse characters who did not portray nurses in the best light. Donelan et al. concluded that the media did not create a permanent negative image of nurses that was harmful to the profession. On the other hand, there were differences between men and women. Women were far more likely to have considered a nursing career than were men. The researchers did not ask the public for their impressions about female nurses and male nurses, just nurses in general. I believe that negative images of male nurses still present in society may be a barrier for men, but *not* for women. I will discuss this more fully later in this chapter.

Minority status

Students with racial and ethnic minority heritages face possible barriers of isolation, cultural insensitivity, and discrimination. Coleman (2008) reported that African American students' sense of isolation was strong. One student said, "I felt like a leper … I felt isolated and intimidated" (p. 10). Wong et al. (2008) reported that African American students had less interaction with their teachers than White classmates. Childs et al. (2004) reviewed several studies that noted the same sense of isolation. Moceri (2010) reported that Hispanic students also felt isolated and discussed the lack of Hispanic nurse role models. Statements of discrimination were also reported by students. One student commented that a teacher said, "Hispanics aren't that smart" (Moceri, 2010, p. 7). Native American students also reported that racism was a problem in their schools (Metz, Cech, Babcock, & Smith, 2011).

Tips for reducing barriers caused by minority status

Battling a sense of isolation is tough for any student. When you feel like an outsider, it becomes difficult to access resources that will help you be successful. Also, isolation can bring on feelings of self-doubt and low self-esteem, which in turn, makes it even more difficult to combat any discrimination. The most important strategy, then, is to take care of any sense of isolation experienced due to race or ethnicity. Getting emotional support from family and from other minority students becomes crucial in helping minority students be successful (Arnault-Pelletier et al., 2006; Childs et al., 2004; Coleman, 2008; Dapremont, 2011; Metz et al., 2011; Moceri, 2010). Dapremont also reported that forming study relationships with White students was also helpful in gaining a sense of belonging. But students benefit from support from teachers and schools also. For example, the University of Saskatchewan and Montana State University have developed comprehensive support programs for Native American students that include academic support (e.g., tutoring, review classes, classes on improving study habits) and social support (e.g., help with housing, finances, childcare, etc.). These programs have reduced the sense of isolation and attrition (Arnault-Pelletier et al., 2006; Metz et al., 2011). Insensitivity and discrimination from teachers can be reduced by sensitivity training for teachers, making sure that the curriculum respects and values other cultures and beliefs, recruiting more minority teachers, and seeking funding to admit more minority students (Childs et al., 2004; Coleman, 2008; Dapremont, 2011). The support program for Native

American students at Montana State University includes helping faculty recognize and reduce biased systems and behaviors (Metz et al., 2011).

Authors also stated that successful minority students report some cultural and personal characteristics that seem to be helpful. Coleman (2008) reported that resiliency, an ability to bounce back and forge ahead, is important. Students said that this resiliency was taught and modeled to them from their families and community leaders. These students also reported that having a strong spiritual side was helpful in facing their barriers. Moceri (2010) reported that Hispanic students talked about having *cabezona*, or an attitude of stubbornness, when they faced barriers. *Cabezona* gives strength and encouragement to keep fighting against injustice. The message here is that minority communities have experience fighting discrimination and other challenges. If you have a minority heritage, use the wisdom of your communities to guide and support you as you battle barriers.

Lack of available jobs

The economic downturn that took hold in 2008 has affected everyone, including nurses. In order to support themselves and their families better, many nurses who had been working part-time started working full time. Some nurses who had planned to retire held on to their jobs instead. Many people who lost their jobs also lost their health insurance. Hospitals and clinics saw a drop in elective surgeries and other medical procedures, but an increase in the number of patients who could not pay their medical bills. This put a financial strain on hospitals and clinics. In order to save money, health care facilities have asked nurses to work more hours and have cut back on hiring new graduate nurses. All of these factors have created a more competitive job market for nurses, especially for new nurses with no experience (Brewer, 2010; Buerhaus, 2009; Gaffney & Rowe, 2011; Malone, Tagliareni, Haney, Taylor, & Mancino, 2010).

The tough job market greatly increases student anxiety. I have seen this anxiety at my own school. A few years ago when jobs for new graduates were more plentiful, students often wanted clinical experiences in many different settings so they could learn a variety of skills. Now, students want clinical experiences they feel will make them more competitive when they hit the job market. This change is wise, but most students don't have a good understanding of what types of clinical experiences will really make them more competitive. For example, I see many students insist on experiences in the intensive care unit (ICU) and emergency department. Students recognize that these clinical settings require nurses to have advanced hospital skills. Students assume that if they have experience in these settings, they will be more competitive in the job market. But this thinking is wrong. Most students do not have enough competence in basic to moderately advanced hospital skills to allow them to move on to advanced skills. Students in these settings may become *exposed* to advanced skills, but are not able to develop *competence* with these skills. Students require much more supervision in these settings, so they cannot practice their nursing independently. Most important, fewer of these settings hire new graduates. Instead, these settings often hire experienced nurses. New graduates usually find jobs in general hospital units and nonhospital settings. Clinical experiences in the intensive care unit or emergency department do not prepare students very well for the places where new graduates usually find their first job. For example, one manager of a general medical unit told me, "Why would I hire a student who has been in the ICU? At best those students have taken care of one or two bedridden patients with a lot of supervision. I want students who have some practice taking care of maybe four patients with just a little supervision. That student will transition more successfully into the employee I need." The important point here is this: be smart! Get as much student experience as you can in the type of clinical setting you *predict* will hire you, not the type of setting you *dream* about hiring you. Once you have gained nursing experience, you will have a better idea of which career direction really speaks to you, and you will be better prepared to pursue that direction.

Anxiety about getting a job has become so high in some students that some requests for clinical experiences have turned into unrealistic demands and ultimatums. For example, I recently had a student in my office very upset that she was assigned to spend six weeks working with the elderly in her first clinical rotation. "How am I going to get a job working with kids?" she cried. "Nobody will hire me if I don't have experience working with kids." It took some time for me to calm her down. She had trouble understanding that nurses have to be trained to work with *all* types of patients, not just patients of their choosing. I told her that she would work with a variety of patients in several different settings while she was in school, including children. She left my office unconvinced and still upset. I later found out that she didn't do well in her clinical. I suspect that her anger and anxiety blinded her from learning. She almost failed the course. I will discuss strategies to help position yourself as best as possible when you look for that first nursing job in Chapter 7.

GENDER-BASED BARRIERS FOR MALE STUDENTS

In the previous section, I reviewed common barriers for all nursing students and strategies that might reduce or prevent these barriers from getting in the way of success. Many of these barriers require students to change behaviors and seek support from family and friends. Also, schools can change practices and make resources available to students that will increase student success. Schools that do this establish a *student-friendly* environment, which creates a win–win situation: students are more successful, schools are able to retain students, and the profession has more new nurses prepared to care for patients of the future.

There are, however, some barriers that are experienced uniquely or more commonly by male students. Most of these barriers come from a long history of patriarchy in our society (see Chapter 3) and nursing's response to patriarchy. This response has supported negative attitudes and discrimination and contributed to an overall sense of role strain for men in nursing. Simpson (2005) described role strain as conflicts that come about as men try to maintain their masculine identities against feminine perceptions and aspects of their jobs. Role strain, on top of the other general barriers, can create a uniquely dangerous level of stress for male nursing students.

That is not to say that female students do not experience gender-based barriers too. However, female students are unlikely to experience gender role strain since nursing is compatible with the feminine gender role in our society. Instead, female students may experience gendered stress by trying to maintain their feminine roles, especially traditional family roles. For example, it is possible that some female students experience conflicts with child care duties at home more frequently than do male students. Unfortunately, there is little research on which barriers are unique to female students. Since modern nursing schools have been dominated by women, it is reasonable to assume that nursing schools, by in large, already provide a *female-friendly* environment. A female-friendly environment supports the needs and preferences of women. If taken too far, a female-friendly environment could become unfriendly to male students. This is why I believe many more men experience gender-based barriers in nursing school than do women. A learning environment that is not friendly to men may contribute to higher attrition rates for male students.

In 2002, the notion of an unfriendly environment for male students caught my attention. It had been 16 years since I graduated from nursing school. In those 16 years, I had seen many changes in gender roles. For example, baby-changing tables are now common in men's public restrooms. Also, I had seen many changes in nursing, including admitting more men in nursing school. In light of these changes, I was very surprised in 2002 to learn that male students at my school were still facing the same gender-related hardships that I had faced 16 years earlier. A male student had asked to meet with me privately to talk about his trouble "fitting in." He told me that he felt that others treated him poorly because he was a man and didn't feel comfortable soothing patients the same way his female classmates did. We talked about this for some time, but I wondered if his male classmates felt the same way. I invited all the male students together one day for lunch and asked them to speak openly about their experiences. I got an earful! Clearly, there were some problems, but were these problems only going on at my school? I wondered if men in other schools were having similar problems. This started my work in researching gender-based barriers for men in nursing school.

At the time, there were a lot of articles written about men's experiences in nursing school. I gathered this information and came up with a list of possible gender-based barriers men face in nursing school. I added a couple of barriers from my own experiences, along with those I heard about from male nurses I knew. In total, I identified 35 possible barriers. From this, I developed a questionnaire and sent it out to 200 male nurses all across the country. I asked these men if they had faced any of these barriers in nursing school, and if they did, did they think these barriers were important. (My assumption was that if men felt a barrier wasn't very important, than it probably was not very stressful.) Over 100 men responded. Their responses indicated that all 35 barriers were present, though it differed from school to school. All of the barriers were considered important by at least some of the men, though most felt that some of the barriers were more important than other barriers. Sadly, the results from men who graduated in the 1970s and 1980s were very similar to those from men that graduated recently. This suggested that conditions in nursing schools had not improved much for men over the past few decades (O'Lynn, 2004).

My research generated a lot of discussion. Many nurse educators began to look at their own programs to see how they might support their male students better. I received requests from across the country and the world for consultation and for permission to use my questionnaire. My research was repeated in a more racially diverse group of male nurses; the results were remarkably similar (Le-Hinds, 2010). Research in Ireland (Keogh & O'Lynn, 2007) found similar barriers for male nursing students there. The same was also found in Canada, England, and Australia (unpublished data).

However, not all the discussion about my research was positive. Some anger was directed at me for criticizing nursing schools. Others denied that barriers for male students were important or that they even existed. One nurse educator even accused me of doctoring my data to push my male agenda! Still today, the topic of how to help men be more successful in nursing schools is controversial. I have been told by both the U.S. Department of Education and a regional health foundation that they would not fund any grants for projects which focus on helping men exclusively, despite the convincing evidence that men (and not women) are in need of support in nursing school. Even in 2011, one graduate student told me that she had an uphill battle convincing her teachers that it was acceptable to research male nursing students. One nurse educator in Illinois told me that her coworkers were very angry that she wanted to explore male gender-based barriers at her school.

It's been 10 years since I started my research on barriers for male nursing students. I continue to explore the topic, but I am cautiously more optimistic today about how men are treated in nursing school. In my travels speaking with students and educators, I hear more positive stories than I heard 10 years ago. But barriers still exist. They aren't experienced by all men at all schools. A certain barrier for one student may be very trivial, yet the same barrier may be very distressing to a different student. More often than not, nurse teachers want to and do provide a supportive environment to all their students, including men. Usually, if present, it is only one or two teachers at a school who might have negative attitudes toward men. Unfortunately, one or two instructors can greatly influence the culture and practices at a nursing school. Their influence could have a negative effect on the potential success of male students; therefore, awareness of male gender-based barriers is important.

In this next section, I will discuss the broad categories of barriers that are unique to or more common to men. Previously, I discussed general barriers in terms of individual factors, school factors, and social/economic factors. These categories don't match the way I think about gender-based barriers; gender-based barriers are too interrelated. In the past, I organized gender-based barriers in terms of those that the school could work on directly and immediately (e.g., teachers making antimale remarks in class) and those

TABLE 5.1 Gender-Based Barriers for Male Nursing Students

Negative View of Men in Nursing

- People important to me did not support my decision to enroll in nursing school.
- As a male, I was not welcomed by most RNs in my clinical rotations.
- My nursing program did not encourage me to strive for leadership roles.
- I felt I had to prove myself in nursing school because people expect nurses to be female.

Feminine Nursing Education

- My nursing program did not include content on men's health issues.
- My nursing program provided few opportunities for classroom debate of issues and concepts.
- My nursing program did not have courses that used competition as a learning incentive.
- Most instructors relied totally on lectures instead of interactive learning activities.
- Most instructors did not allow group or teamwork on assignments.
- My nursing program did not prepare me well for working with mostly female coworkers.

Lack of Role Models/Isolationism

- Before nursing school, I never knew a male nurse.
- Before nursing school, no one I knew ever had care from a male nurse.
- My nursing program did not actively recruit male students to enroll.
- There were no male teachers at my nursing school.
- There were no other male students in my class.
- My nursing program did not teach about men's roles in the history of nursing.
- I did not get to work with male nurses in my clinical rotations.
- I was not encouraged to contact other male students for support.
- I was not invited to participate in all student activities.
- My nursing program did not have a male mentorship program.
- I felt isolated from other men at my school since I was a nursing student.

Antimale Language

- Most of my instructors referred to the nurse as "she."
- Most of my textbooks/readings referred to the nurse as "she."
- There were times in class when my instructors made disparaging remarks against men.
- In lectures, men were portrayed as the perpetrators of crimes, and rarely the victims.

Different Treatment

- In my nursing program, male students were usually used when instructors wanted to demonstrate assessment of the chest and/or pelvic areas.
- During my obstetric (mother–baby) rotation, I had different requirements or limitations placed on me compared to my female classmates.
- In my nonobstetric rotations, I was usually assigned to care for male patients.
- In my nursing program, male and female students were treated differently by the instructors more than I had originally anticipated.

Communication

- My nursing program did not discuss communication challenges between men and women and how to overcome them for good teamwork and nursing care.
- My gender was a barrier in developing collegial relationships with some of my instructors.

(continued)

TABLE 5.1   Gender-Based Barriers for Male Nursing Students (*continued*)

Touch/Feminine Caring

- My instructors did not give me much guidance, as a man, on the appropriate use of touch.
- My instructors emphasized caring behaviors that I think are feminine.
- My instructors did not discuss or demonstrate masculine caring behaviors.
- I was nervous women would accuse me of sexual inappropriateness when I touched their bodies.

Source: Adapted from the Inventory of Male Friendliness in Nursing Schools, O'Lynn (2003/2004).

that the school could not fix directly (e.g., family not supporting the male student's decision to go to nursing school). Over the past couple of years, I've come to realize that schools have much greater influence on the nursing profession and society than I had thought. Nursing schools prepare the nurses and leaders of the profession of tomorrow. These nurses and leaders will shape the practices and expectations of the profession, and how society will view nurses and the profession.

Schools must take the lead in reducing gender-based barriers and the stress that these barriers cause male students. That is not to say that you don't need to act also. Just like with general barriers for nursing students, you will need to work on reducing the gender barriers in your own lives. It is my hope, however, that your actions will encourage your school to become more *male-friendly*. In doing so, I believe there will be a balance struck between a female-friendly *and* a male-friendly school environment so that a student's sex and gender have no bearing on the learning environment.

I group the gender barriers by theme: negative view of men in nursing; feminine nursing education; lack of role models; antimale language; different treatment; communication; and touch/feminine caring. (The last two, communication and touch/feminine caring, are so important that I have devoted a separate chapter to each of these.) Table 5.1 lists the individual barriers from the questionnaire and how they are grouped into these themes, although some barriers could be included under more than one theme. Let's look at these barriers more closely.

Negative View of Men in Nursing

In Chapter 3, I discussed how nursing has become dominated by women and how society's ideas about masculinity has steered men away from nursing. Obviously, men in nursing school, such as yourselves, have moved past these negative ideas; otherwise, they (and you) would not have chosen to apply to nursing school in the first place. However, these ideas may still influence family members, friends, and even teachers. The lack of support and understanding from these important people create a barrier unique to men; unique in the sense that women get fewer, if any, messages that nursing is not appropriate for them because they are women.

One barrier that continues to creep up for some men in nursing is the fear that others will think they are gay because they want to be nurses

(Bartfay, Bartfay, Clow, & Wu, 2010; Dyck, Oliffe, Phinney, & Garrett, 2009; Hart, 2005; Haywood, 1994; Kelly, Shoemaker, & Steele, 1996; Lo & Brown, 1999; Wilson, 2005). Of course, there is no problem being gay, but if a student is *not* gay, it may be upsetting for him to be labeled as gay since there is much antigay prejudice still present in our society. This fear about being mislabeled speaks to beliefs about masculinity and how one's masculinity may be called into question for wanting to pursue a profession dominated by women. This fear is so strong in some male nurses that they go out of their way to let people know that they are not gay, or they show that they are still masculine in appearance and behavior (Dyck et al., 2009; Tillman & Machtmes, 2008). This creates a problem for everyone. First, the man who is fearful has conflict with his career choice, which may lead to self-doubt and stress. And second, this fear sends a negative message about male nurses who are gay or about those who might display feminine characteristics, as if to say, "I'm not one of *those* kinds of nurses." This type of message contradicts the values of the nursing profession and only worsens negative stereotypes. (I have not seen anything written that suggests that female students fear being labeled as lesbian simply because they are nurses. This barrier is unique to male students.)

I did not include the fear of being mislabeled as gay as a barrier on my questionnaire because sexuality is complicated. If a gay male nursing student experiences discrimination, is it because he is a man in nursing, is it because he is gay, or is it both? In my research, I wanted to focus only on being a man in nursing, so I left sexuality out of my questionnaire. I have not seen any research that explored whether or not men in nursing are more likely to be gay than in other professions, probably because whether or not a nurse is gay has no bearing on his ability to be a good nurse. Still, the fear of being perceived as gay and antigay discrimination is important, and may lead to much stress for some male nursing students, especially if it leads to negative thoughts from the student's family and friends.

Even worse, a horrible stereotype that won't seem to go away is that some people wonder if men enter nursing because they are sexual predators who want to have access to potential victims. Unfortunately, today's media have worsened this stereotype (Bartfay et al., 2010; Evans, 2002). Stories of men who molest or rape children and other vulnerable victims are sensationalized and shown over and over again in today's 24-hour media environment. Television shows such as *America's Most Wanted* and *Nancy Grace* give viewers every graphic and horrible detail about these crimes. Due to the constant exposure, some people may think that these crimes are on the rise. Stories about teachers and health care workers who prey on their students or patients are especially troubling because these workers are trusted and held to high standards. To make matters worse, some nurse administrators and leaders feed into the stereotype by claiming that men should be viewed suspiciously (Cude & Winfrey, 2007; Salvage, 2000; Hawke, 1998). The increased attention has taken a toll on male nursing students. In my research on gender barriers, men who went to nursing school in the 1970s and 1980s generally were not concerned about false sexual accusations from their patients, with only 27.5% saying that this barrier was a factor for them.

More recent graduates were far more concerned; 45.2% reported this barrier (O'Lynn, 2003). Kermode (2006) also noted that the students he interviewed complained that men were continuously portrayed as violent abusers. Male students found this insulting.

The view others have of men in nursing is important. If your family members and friends tease you about your decision to become a nurse or try to convince you to change majors, a valuable support system may be out of your reach (Bartfay et al., 2010; Wilson, 2005). If others look at you with suspicion, you may feel like you have to walk on eggshells. Over half of the men surveyed by my Irish colleague and me reported that they felt they had to prove themselves in nursing school simply because they were men, and over 75% of men felt that this barrier was important (Keogh & O'Lynn, 2007). What they had to prove probably varied from man to man, but based on the gendered barriers they described, they may have had to prove that they were morally fit and not sexual predators, and that they were just as caring and qualified as female nurses. This need to prove one's character can be a great weight on the shoulders of male students.

In Chapter 3, I discussed why some women in nursing don't want more men to enter the field. Some believe that nursing should remain female-dominated in order to balance out a male-dominated health care system (Ryan & Porter, 1993). Others fear that if a large number of men become nurses, nursing will lose many of its positive characteristics that have been developed by women (Evans, 1997; Ryan & Porter, 1993; Williams, 2001). Still others fear that men will advance their nursing careers by taking advantage of the privileges men have in our society and, once men are in power, try to dominate female nurses (Evans, 1997; Williams, 2001; Wilson, 2005). Ryan and Porter stated that men who enter nursing should "do so on [women's] nursing's terms" (p. 267). These attitudes lead to a very unwelcoming environment for men. Some teachers, nurses, and classmates can give you a cold shoulder for no other reason than you are male. In their minds, as a man, you are a member of an enemy group that will damage nursing.

Fortunately, I believe these attitudes are melting away. More and more nurses understand the benefit of a diverse workforce. I believe most nurses welcome all talented newcomers regardless of sex and gender, even though nursing may not yet know how to integrate diversity as smoothly as it should. There are still a few nurses with old-fashioned attitudes about men in nursing who may still give the cold shoulder. A problem for nursing students, however, is that these nurses with negative attitudes may be your teachers. A few studies suggest that nursing instructors are slower than staff nurses and patients to adopt positive attitudes about men in nursing (Cude & Winfrey, 2007; McRae, 2003), maybe because some nursing instructors don't work much in clinical settings. Change is common in clinical settings, but less so in nursing schools. Nursing schools can be rather isolated to themselves, and some negative nurse teachers may exercise great control over the curriculum and culture within a school. Another thought is that nurses who are passionate about teaching the old-fashioned ways of nursing find their way into education roles. Still another thought is that there are very few men working as nursing instructors, only about 5% of full-time nursing teachers

(National League of Nursing, 2011c). Working with more men as cowork-ers may wash away negative stereotypes about male nurses (McRae, 2003; McMillan, Morgan, & Arment, 2006). With little exposure to male nurses and male coworkers, some negative nurse teachers never learn the positive influ-ence men make on nursing. Regardless of the reasons, male nursing students continue to report receiving the cold shoulder from some of their female teachers (Kermode, 2006).

Tips on reducing the negative image of men in nursing

My most important tip here is to speak up; be as vocal as you can be about men in nursing. I believe accurate information is the best weapon against negative images and the prejudice those images might create. When someone says something to you about men in nursing that is not right, take the oppor-tunity to educate them. Tell them that men have been nurses for centuries and have done much to make nursing what it is today. Let them know that nurses are highly trained lifesavers. Nurses have excellent problem-solving skills, are able to think fast on their feet, and fight for the needs of patients in an unfriendly health care system. Let them know that nursing is neither women's or men's work, but instead, nursing is tough physical and emotional *human* work. As more people get to know your fine qualities, they will start to attach those qualities to their ideas about male nurses.

I have three other recommendations. First, fight negative images of male nurses in the media and entertainment industries. Write letters of complaint to studios, television producers, and publishers who portray male nurses negatively. Let them know how their images harm men in nursing and the patients they serve. Let them know how their work harms you personally. The media and entertainment industries do listen to their audiences, espe-cially when enough people complain. Second, make yourself visible as a nursing student or nurse, especially to young people. Visit schools, churches, and youth groups for health fairs, career fairs, or classes. Write articles or make short videos for kids about men in nursing. An excellent example is the work of Maggie Dorsey. Although not a male nurse herself, Dr. Dorsey wrote a childrens book titled *My Hero, My Dad the Nurse* (Dorsey, 2008). This book teaches children the appropriateness and honor of nursing for men. Young people are very impressionable. If you present yourself and other men as nurses and role models, you have an opportunity to create a new and posi-tive image of male nurses in the minds of these young people. And third, encourage your female peers to pursue their career dreams. Reassure them that your own actions to seek skill, knowledge, and career advancement do not come at their expense. Nursing has plenty of opportunities for anyone, male or female, who is willing to work hard and advance their educations. Applaud their accomplishments and the value they bring to nursing.

Feminine Nursing Education

Nightingale established the model for the modern nursing school based on the assumption that only women should be educated as nurses. For much of the early 20th century, most schools did not allow men to enroll (Kalisch & Kalisch,

2004). In schools that did accept men, men were kept away from the female students and were not offered some classes, such as obstetrics. More women took teaching positions in nursing schools as schools freed themselves from under the control of patriarchal hospital and legal systems. Female teachers, by in large, determined how students would be taught. Over time, nursing programs developed school cultures that catered to the needs and preferences of female teachers and female students.

Feminist approaches to teaching and learning began to infuse nursing schools as the feminist movement took hold in society in the latter half of the 20th century. Feminism comes in many shapes and forms, some of which have been accepted or fallen out of favor over time (see Chapter 3). Individual schools and individual teachers may follow different versions of feminism to match their individual beliefs. I believe, however, that two important authors have shaped much of the feminist influence in schools of nursing: Gilligan and Carper.

Gilligan (1982) studied how men and women differ when they make ethical decisions. In a nutshell, Gilligan noted that men tend to follow a pattern that she called an *ethics of justice*. This pattern encourages the person to focus on what is right and wrong, what is just and unjust, what is fair. Women, on the other hand, follow a pattern she called an *ethics of care*. This pattern encourages the person to explore compromise and recognize the other's humanness in order to keep relationships positive. A sense of fairness becomes less important than a sense of positive connection with others. Gilligan's work has been both criticized and supported over the years. Nevertheless, many in nursing adopted Gilligan's basic assumption because it matches their beliefs that women are better suited for caring roles than are men.

Carper (1978) also noted important differences between men and women, not in their ethics, but rather in how they gain and use knowledge. Carper suggested that men tend to rely on the scientific method to build knowledge. This method emphasizes the use of objective, nonemotional data, whereas women tend to use data from multiple sources including their personal knowledge, values, and the arts. Many call these multiple types of knowledge women's ways of knowing. This phrase bothers me since it implies that men don't use these types of knowledge, when in fact, men do use them. Nursing has embraced the work of Carper so completely that Carper's women's ways of knowing have become a mainstay in many nursing schools.

Neither Gilligan nor Carper suggested that *all* men and *all* women follow these patterns. Instead, there are tendencies for men and women to use these patterns unless they are forced or guided to use a different pattern. Some feminist scholars in nursing have used the works of Gilligan and Carper (and others) to highlight the differences between men and women. These nurse scholars have used the nursing education system to help new nurses and researchers increase the use of women's ways in order to balance what they believe to be a masculine health care system (e.g., Arslanian-Engoren, 2002; Chapman, 1997; Kvigne & Kirkevold, 2002).

Although this effort is beneficial to nursing, a problem occurs when a school emphasizes the ways of women so much so that the value of diversity is ignored. This sets up a biased setting that some men find hypocritical and troubling. Not much research has been done on this topic. In my own research, I did not ask men directly about a feminist bias. Instead, I asked men about situations that might stem from a feminist bias in their programs. For example, over half of the men reported that the history of men in nursing was not presented in school and that men's health issues were ignored. Other barriers identified by the men included hearing antimale remarks in class, referring to nurses as "she," being treated differently than female classmates, the lack of recruitment of men into the nursing program, and no encouragement of men to pursue leadership roles in class. Other researchers have confirmed a feminine and/or feminist culture to nursing school (Dyck et al., 2009; Ellis, Meeker, & Hyde, 2006; Kermode, 2006; Lo & Brown, 1999; Stott, 2007).

Sometimes, bias is visible in how teachers teach and the classroom environments they create. For example, Stott (2007) reported that men need to feel independent with their studying and not micromanaged by their teachers. Ellis et al. (2006) noted that male students became frustrated with excessive reflections and talking things out. Kermode (2006) reported that men said that feminist views were "in," and that men were not valued. Also, nursing students, *both male and female*, reported more feminist bias in their school than did students from nonnursing schools. Dyck et al. (2009) observed that male students were more willing to challenge their teachers than female students. This masculine pattern of debate fed the idea that male students were troublemakers. These students also reported frustration at the female teachers' emphasis on talking about relationships and feelings when it slowed down the efficiency of the class. Male students also reported that their teachers assumed that all students were familiar with female anatomy and experiences when many of the men were not familiar. Paterson et al. (1996) reported that male students didn't feel that female teachers understood them as men.

Despite this, the desire by some to keep feminism in nursing continues to be expressed. Chapman (1997) recommended that nursing schools should adopt feminist structures in order to combat a patriarchal health system. He stated, "…male teachers of female student nurses should be prepared to study feminism, feminine ways of knowing, and feministic knowledge. The feministic approach is unlikely to harm male students" (p. 213). I wouldn't go as far as Chapman. Total exclusion of other belief systems in favor of feminism leads to tunneled vision and lack of respect for diverse viewpoints. Exclusion of other belief systems can create an unfriendly school environment for male students.

Tips on facing feminine nursing education

My advice to you here is to embrace the opportunity to learn new ideas. Look at it this way: if you were taking an art class and the teacher said not to use any blue or green, but only paint in red and yellow, your artistic options would be limited. Similarly, you will be limited in your ability as nurses if you reject feminism outright or anything else you perceive as feminine. Be open to learning about and understanding these viewpoints. This will allow you to see the complexities and humanness of others, including your patients. Also, be open to recognizing the reality of patriarchy and how it hurts both women *and* men.

This is *not* to say that you must abandon your own beliefs or your own masculinity. If you feel that comments in class are disrespectful to you, speak up. If the teacher has an approach that isn't in line with how you learn, meet with the teacher and discuss ways to help you learn better. Men and women have much to learn from each other. Masculine and feminine approaches to knowledge, to care, or to relationships have benefits and challenges— neither is superior over the other. Your goal should be to learn how to look at a situation from multiple angles and become well versed in using multiple approaches to solve problems. Help female teachers and classmates improve their abilities to see issues from multiple perspectives as well. Share your perspectives on issues from a masculine perspective. Request that class discussions be safe spaces to air multiple viewpoints. Improving your ability to listen respectfully to others' perspectives and to ask others to listen respectfully to your perspectives will build excellent teamwork and nursing care skills.

The Lack of Role Models and Isolation

Multiple studies have reported that male nursing students have complained about a lack of role models over the years (e.g., Kelly et al., 1996; Okrainec, 1994; Stott, 2007; Streubert, 1994). As I noted earlier, few nursing schools include content about the history of men in nursing (which is why I included Chapter 2 in this book). Without the knowledge of men's historical past, some people think that men are a recent intruder into nursing. Worse, there are few male nurses who serve as modern day role models on a national level. Although there are more men in nursing school today than when I went to nursing school (13% of all students in 2010 [National League for Nursing, 2011d]), different schedules may separate men from each other. Also, only about 5% of full-time teachers in nursing school are men (National League for Nursing, 2011c). In my earlier research, 67.8% of all the men surveyed said they had no male teachers at their school, and 62.7% said they never had the opportunity to work with male nurses in their clinical rotations (O'Lynn, 2004). Still today, I am the only man of some 22 full-time teachers at my school of nursing.

The lack of role models and male classmates can lead some men to feel isolated. Stott (2007) reported that isolation was a common complaint from the men she studied. These men reported fear of speaking up when they were in the minority. One student said, "You learn to bite your tongue because you don't want to be shot down in flames by a group of women... they can be very intimidating in some respects" (p. 328). Bell-Scriber (2008) also reported that the men she interviewed felt isolated, which led them to feel like they didn't blend in or belong.

Tips on facing isolation

My advice is to connect with other men, both past and present. First, reflect on the men highlighted in Chapter 2. Think about the values that made them exceptional nurses. Adopt these values in your own work as a nurse and you will be admired and successful. Second, connect with other male nurses and male classmates. Some schools offer men's groups (Wilson, 2005). These groups allow men to meet, discuss issues, and learn from each other. Connecting with other men helps you feel that you are not alone. I facilitated a men's group for a couple of years. We met over lunch once a semester. At the meetings, I invited a male nurse working in the local area to join us. Some of these nurses were staff nurses, some were managers, and some were nurse specialists. The students appreciated hearing about their experiences and the advice they gave the students. I think most of all, the students enjoyed the opportunity to have a men's only social time. If your school doesn't offer a men's group, then start one. It can be informal—meet for pizza or go to a sporting event, or ask a teacher to facilitate a group for you. For some of you, a local chapter of the American Assembly for Men in Nursing (AAMN) may be available in your area. AAMN is a nursing organization with the goals of bringing more men into nursing, offering professional development and mentorship opportunities, and addressing men's health issues. Involvement with AAMN allows you to connect to men from other schools and male nurse leaders both locally and nationally. Third, and perhaps most important, advocate to spend time with male nurses in your clinical rotations. Working side-by-side with a male nurse is the best way to learn how men do the work of nursing. Paterson et al. (1996) reported that male students learned how to care as men by observing male nurses. These students noted important differences between how men and women care for patients, and that these differences were never discussed by their female teachers or classmates. Clearly not all nursing care differs between men and women. For example, the technique for giving an insulin shot is the same whether the nurse is male or female. But other actions have more apparent differences, such as how the nurse communicates with patients or how the nurse provides comfort (see Chapter 6). Whenever possible, ask to be paired up with a male nurse in your senior practicum or capstone experience. (This rotation, done just before you graduate, has you work side-by-side with a staff nurse for an extended period of time.) Observe how this male nurse cares for his patients. When paired with a male nurse, feel free to discuss gender differences with him and with your teachers. Think about how he works with others and solves problems. Allow him to guide your developing style of nursing care.

Gender-Biased Language and Imagery

Today, most language has become gender-neutral. For example, *police officer* has replaced *policeman* since many officers are now women. In health care, it is rare to hear the term *lady doctor*. Instead, the word *doctor* brings up an image of either a male or female doctor. The same cannot be said for the word *nurse*. Since relatively few men are nurses, the image for nurse is usually feminine in people's minds. This feminine image leads people to use the word "she" when referring to the generic nurse. For example, "The nurse should display empathy. *She* should always keep in mind what the illness means to the patient." Kelly et al. (1996) reported that male students find this feminine pronoun bothersome, as if it were a constant reminder that men do not belong in nursing. Bell-Scriber (2008) reported that the male students she interviewed found the use of "she" to be noticeable, which reinforced their minority status. In my own research, I noted that 82% of men reported that their textbooks used the word "she" for nurse (O'Lynn, 2004); however, the men did not report that this issue was as important as some of the other barriers they faced. In other words, men found this problem to be irritating, but not significant. Similarly, Smith (2006) noted that older male nursing students did not find the feminine imagery and language too bothersome because they "had faced larger problems and were not going to let these issues affect their success" (p. 267).

Nevertheless, the constant use of feminine language and images for nursing over time does lead to a sense of exclusion. Feminine language and images become a major symbol for nursing. Symbols are important. Symbols create a bond of collegiality. If symbols are overwhelmingly feminine, men may feel uncomfortable and discounted (Sullivan, 2000). The AAMN has suggested that the use of feminine language and images goes against the values of the nursing profession and is disrespectful to men. They further noted that the use of feminine language is hypocritical to the feminist position of using gender-neutral language for occupations that were or are male-dominated. The AAMN described nurse teachers as role models and leaders for future generations of nurses. As such, teachers should be particularly careful not to exclude any student by using feminine language or imagery. The AAMN passed a resolution at its 2011 annual meeting challenging nursing schools to take the lead in reducing exclusive language and images (Lecher, 2011).

Tips for facing feminine language and imagery

In my experience, nursing textbooks have become much better in using gender-neutral language and including pictures of male nurses and minority nurses. Instead, the issue is more common with teachers and nurses using the word "she" inappropriately. Often, these teachers and nurses are older, so maybe old habits do die hard. My advice is to speak up when feminine language or images are used inappropriately. Do not interrupt the person, but rather speak to the person later about their noninclusive language. The purpose here is to raise awareness, not to criticize.

For example, in a recent staff meeting, a coworker was planning a "Student-Preceptor Tea," a gathering designed for junior students to meet with senior students to thank them for working with them. Light refreshments were going to be served at the tea. I had concerns about the event's title. In America, men do not usually go to teas. Images of hats, flowers, and pretty teapots and teacups came to my mind. I spoke to my coworkers later that the image of the tea was not gender-neutral. Male students may not choose to attend this event. Since the event was not going to include a formal tea ceremony, why not call the event "Student-Preceptor Social"? My coworker agreed and changed the name of the event.

Differential Treatment

A common theme in articles written about male nursing students is how they are treated differently than their female classmates. Most authors used reports from male nursing students, rather than witnessing actual differences in treatment. Some of the reported differences may seem minor to some. For example, one of the students interviewed by Stott (2007) reported that, as a male, he was the student asked to remove his shirt in class so that others could see how to do a procedure or give a urine sample for the class to examine. Wilson (2005) reported similar complaints. This may be upsetting for some students, but for others, it might only be a minor irritation. Other differences are more significant. For example, male students have reported that patients sometimes refuse care from them simply because they are male (Paterson et al, 1996; Smith, 2006; Stott, 2007; Wilson, 2005). Teachers rarely discuss this issue with male students, even though students need guidance on how to work through this difficult situation (Paterson et al., 1996). Other differences include being asked to care for or assist with more difficult patients because these patients required physical strength, being assigned to care for only male patients, or being discouraged from certain specialties such as women's health or pediatrics, or not getting as much attention in clinical rotations as do female students (Bell-Scriber, 2008; Cude & Winfrey, 2007; Hart, 2005; Kelly et al., 1996; Milligan, 2001).

Perhaps most important was Bell-Scriber's (2008) study in which she interviewed teachers and students at a nursing school, as well as attended some classes and observed how teachers responded to male students. Bell-Scriber noted that the men felt that the teachers were harsher with them than their female classmates. Sometimes the teacher had an angry tone or had body language that communicated disapproval. One of the female classmates agreed with the men, noting that teachers picked on the male students. In the classroom, Bell-Scriber observed a cooler climate for the men than for the women. A cooler climate might occur for many different reasons, but one reason may be outright prejudice against men. Bell-Scriber's most distressing finding came from interviewing the teachers. One teacher said:

> It seems to me … it's always the males who are whispering or condescending. I think a lot of the males I experience that go into nursing; they're going into it for the wrong reasons. Whatever they wanted to do didn't work out. And they have more of a chip on their shoulder, a confrontational attitude. Like we have something to prove ourselves or something. (p. 147)

When questioned further, this teacher said that she would like to get rid of all the male students. Another teacher interviewed said that some of the teachers at that school didn't know what to do with male students, and that some thought the male students were lazy. Clearly, if you had any of these teachers, you could easily see how you might be treated differently than your female classmates.

Tips on facing differential treatment

I believe the teachers interviewed by Bell-Scriber (2008) are uncommon. Although I did hear once about a teacher who bragged that she never allowed a male student to pass her classes (she was later sued and lost her teaching position), my recent experience has been that most teachers are very welcoming to male students. This is good news, and news to keep in mind.

Sometimes a teacher's behavior can be misinterpreted. Recently, I met with a student who complained that I was impatient with her in clinical. She believed I thought she was a poor student and was afraid that she would fail the class. I was surprised by this because I considered her a very good student. After a long discussion about the specifics, I became aware that my body language communicated impatience and negativity. The student used my behavior when I watched her listen to a patient's heart and lungs as an example. The student observed that I had my arms crossed, I had a sour look on my face, and I left the room quickly after watching her. As it turns out, I crossed my arms to prevent my lab coat from getting in the way of the student's work as I leaned over the bed. My nonsmiling face was actually a facial expression of me concentrating on what the student was doing. I left the room quickly because I had another student waiting. We both learned a lot from this discussion. The student learned not to assume the worst when interpreting body language, and I learned to take a few seconds after observing the student and praise her on her performance.

My point here is this: sometimes our interpretations are inaccurate, but sometimes they might be dead-on. If you believe you are being treated differently because you are a man, you must speak up. Check in with other male students, and even your female classmates. Do they have the same perceptions as you? If they do, you may feel validated that something is going on. If they do not, this is an opportunity for you to reflect on why you have these perceptions. Then, meet with the teacher, the nurse, or the classmate and share your perceptions with her or him. This will allow the other person an opportunity to resolve any misconceptions and become more aware of their own behavior. For this to be successful, be sure to share specific examples. Vague comments like "I feel like you ignore me" will not help the other person understand your point of view. Usually, a heart-to-heart talk will improve the situation. If not, then plan a meeting with your advisor or with an administrator.

Gender bias and differential treatment are unacceptable and must be brought to the attention of others. Unfortunately, my experience with male students is that many of them are hesitant to speak up. Many choose to suffer in silence. Some students assume that speaking up will do no good, or worse, that speaking up will only cause the teacher to retaliate. But staying silent does nothing to resolve the problem. I was surprised by the male silence at my school. Recently, the dean and I met with the male students over breakfast. We wanted to check in with them and see if there were any gender issues they were experiencing. Overall, we were pleased to hear that the men were doing well and had no concerns except one: female bullying. Some of the male students were growing quite concerned about how some of their female classmates were bullying each other. The men didn't know how to address this problem, but wanted the problem taken care of because it was bringing down student morale. One said, "I don't want to get in the middle of a cat fight between the women." The men noted that women fight differently than men. They didn't know how to break up the fights. Also, the men reported that this problem had been going on for some time. When I asked them why they hadn't mentioned it to someone before, there was a dead silence in the room. Perhaps the men didn't know how to report the problem or to whom. Perhaps the men didn't think the problem could be resolved. Perhaps the men needed to be in the company of other men, a friendly audience to report the problem. Regardless, they did speak up that day. Now the school has implemented activities to bring the issue of bullying out in the open. This might not have happened if the men had not spoken up.

SUMMARY

I'm not someone who usually talks about "how bad I got it" as an explanation for not meeting my goals. On the other hand, sometimes the playing field just isn't level. Researchers and nurse scholars have studied men's experiences in nursing school for decades and have come up with the same general conclusion: men have it tougher in nursing school than women. There is no doubt about it. First, men experience the possible barriers faced by *all* nursing students. These include barriers internal to the student (e.g., poor study habits and poor coping skills) and external to the student (e.g., school schedules and a tight job market). These general barriers can prevent any student from getting the most out of their nursing education. In addition, men, and not women, face unique gender-based barriers in nursing school that come from a long history of patriarchy and prejudice against men in nursing. These gender-based barriers add an extra layer of stress on male students, which may account for higher attrition rates for male nursing students. In effect, these extra barriers can be just enough to boot some men off the nursing school island.

Fortunately, the intensity of these barriers is dropping in most settings. Slowly, men are becoming more accepted in nursing, and nursing schools are changing. However, the changes are happening slowly in some places. Many men report that they hardly face any gender-based barriers; instead they struggle with many of the same barriers experienced by their female classmates. I believe most men are feeling welcomed and supported. Still, other men report they face terrible gender barriers, even though those barriers may come from just a few teachers, nurses, classmates, or family members and friends. For these men, I hope for courage, endurance, and success in their journeys.

In this chapter, I have discussed common barriers for male nursing students. I believe having more awareness of these barriers is necessary to fight barriers early, before barriers get out of hand. I have also provided some tips for addressing barriers. These tips come from my own experiences and observations with students, as well as the experiences and observations of others. There may be other tips I didn't mention. Some of you will come up with approaches to fight barriers that work in your own particular situations. I encourage you to problem-solve and find new ways. If you find a different approach that works, share it with others; the more tips that are available to men, the greater the chances that all men will overcome gender-based barriers. Perhaps, in just a few short years, men's gender-based barriers will become something of nursing's history and never again need discussion in a book such as this.

REFERENCES

Aiken, L. H., Clarke, S. P., Cheung, R. B., Sloane, D. M., & Silas, J. H. (2003). Educational levels of hospital nurses and surgical patient mortality. *JAMA, 290*, 1617–1623.

Alcohol & Drug Abuse Weekly. (2006). Lawsuit seeks to repeal financial aid drug exclusion. *Alcohol & Drug Abuse Weekly, 18*(18), 4–5.

American Association of Colleges of Nursing [AACN]. (2010). *Tri-Council for Nursing issues new consensus policy statement on the educational advancement of registered nurses.* Retrieved from http://www.aacn.nche.edu

American Association of Colleges of Nursing [AACN]. (2011). *Nursing faculty shortage.* Retrieved from http://www.aacn.nche.edu/Media/FactSheets/FacultyShortage.htm

Arnault-Pellitier, V., Brown, S., Desjarlais, J., & McBeth, B. (2006). Circle of strength. *Canadian Nurse, 102*(4), 22–26.

Arslanian-Engoren, C. (2002). Feminist poststructuralism: A methodological paradigm for examining clinical decision-making. *Journal of Advanced Nursing, 37*(6), 512–517.

Assessment Technologies Institute. (2011). Home page. Retrieved from http://www.atitesting.com

Bartfay, W. J., Bartfay, E., Clow, K. A., & Wu, T. (2010). Attitudes and perceptions towards men in nursing education. *The Internet Journal of Allied Health Sciences and Practice, 8*(2), ISSN 1540-580X.

Bell-Scriber, M. J. (2008). Warming the nursing education climate for traditional age learners who are male. *Nursing Education Perspectives, 29*(3), 143–150.

Boley, P., & Whitney, K. (2003). Grade disputes: Considerations for nursing faculty. *Journal of Nursing Education, 42*(5), 198–203.

Boyd, M. A. (2002). Stress management and crisis intervention. In M. A. Boyd (Ed.). *Psychiatric nursing: Contemporary practice* (2nd ed., pp. 920–948). Philadelphia: Lippincott.

Brewer, S. (2010). Landing a job in a tough economy. *Lippincott's 2010 Nursing Career Directory.* Ambler, PA: Lippincott.

Buerhaus, P. I. (2009). The shape of the recovery: Economic implications for the nursing workforce. *Nursing Economics, 27*(5), 336, 338–340.

Campbell, A. R., & Dickson, C. J. (1996). Predicting student success: A 10-year review using integrative review and meta-analysis. *Journal of Professional Nursing, 12*(1), 47–59.

Carper, B. A. (1978). Fundamental patterns of knowing in nursing. *Advances in Nursing Science, 1*(1), 13–24.

Chapman, E. (1997). Nurse education: A feminist approach. *Nurse Education Today, 17*, 209–214.

Chee, M. W. L., & Chuah, L. Y. M. (2008). Functional neuroimaging insights into how sleep and sleep deprivation affect memory and cognition. *Current Opinion in Neurology, 21*(4), 417–423.

Chickering, A. W., & Gamson, Z. F. (1987). Seven principles for good practice in undergraduate education. *American Association for Higher Education (AAHE) Bulletin, 39*(7), 3–7.

Childs, G., Jones, R., Nugent, K. E., & Cook, P. (2004). Retention of African-American students in baccalaureate nursing programs: Are we doing enough? *Journal of Professional Nursing, 20*(2), 129–133.

Clark, C. M., & Springer, P. J. (2007). Incivility in nursing education: A descriptive study of definitions and prevalence. *Journal of Nursing Education, 46*(1), 7–14.

Coleman, L. D. (2008). Experiences of African American students in a predominantly White, two-year nursing program. *ABNF Journal, 19*(1), 8–13.

Crowell, D. M. (2011). *Complexity leadership: Nursing's role in health care delivery.* Philadelphia: F. A. Davis.

Cude, G., & Winfrey, K. (2007). The hidden barrier: Gender bias: Fact or fiction? *AWHONN, 11*(3), 254–265.

Daley, B. J., Shaw, C. R., Balistrieri, T., Glassenapp, K., & Piacentine, L. (1999). Concept maps: A strategy to teach and evaluate critical thinking. *Journal of Nursing Education, 38*, 42–47.

Dapremont, J. A. (2011). Success in nursing school: Black nursing students' perception of peers, family, and faculty. *Journal of Nursing Education, 50*(5), 254–260.

Deary, I. J., Watson, R., & Hogston, R. (2003). A longitudinal cohort study of burnout and attrition in nursing students. *Journal of Advanced Nursing, 43*(1), 71–81.

Donelan, K., Buerhaus, P., DesRoches, C., Dittus, R., & Dutwin, D. (2008). Public perceptions of nursing careers: The influence of the media and shortages. *Nursing Economics, 26*(3), 143–165.

Dorsey, M. T. (2008). *My hero, my dad the nurse.* Retrieved from http://www.usca.edu/myheromydadthenurse/

Drill, H. (2010). So, you need college financial aid? *PN, 64*(11), 22–23.

Dunham, K. S. (2001). *How to survive nursing school and maybe even love nursing school! A guide for students.* Philadelphia: F. A. Davis.

Dyck, J. M., Oliffe, J., Phinney, A., & Garrett, B. (2009). Nursing instructors' and male nursing students' perceptions of undergraduate, classroom nursing education. *Nurse Education Today, 29*, 649–653.

Ellis, D. M., Meeker, B. J., & Hyde, B. L. (2006). Exploring men's perceived educational experiences in a baccalaureate program. *Journal of Nursing Education, 45*(12), 523–527.

Evans, J. (1997). Men in nursing: Issues of gender segregation and hidden advantage. *Journal of Advanced Nursing, 26*(2), 226–231.

Evans, J. (2002). Cautious caregivers: Gender stereotypes and the sexualization of men nurses' touch. *Journal of Advanced Nursing, 40*(4), 441–448.

Fowles, E. R. (1992). Predictors of success on NCLEX-RN and within the nursing curriculum: Implications for early intervention. *Journal of Nursing Education, 31*, 53–57.

Gaffney, T. A., & Rowe, D. (2011). Navigating a competitive job market. *Imprint, 58*(1), 49–53.

Gilligan, C. (1982). *In a different voice: Psychological theory and women's development.* Cambridge, MA: Harvard University Press.

Gordon, S. (2005). Nursing against the odds: *How health care cost-cutting, media stereotypes, and medical hubris undermine nursing and patient care.* New York: Cornell University Press.

Halbach, M. M., Spann, C. O., & Egan, G. (2003). Effect of sleep deprivation on medical resident and student cognitive function: A prospective study. *American Journal of Obstetrics & Gynecology, 188*(5), 1198–1201.

Hart, K. A. (2005). What do men in nursing really think? *Nursing 2005, 35*(11), 46–48.

Hawke, C. (1998). Nursing a fine line: Patient privacy and sex discrimination. *Nursing Management, 29*(10), 56–61.

Haywood, M. (1994). Male order. *Nursing Times, 90*(20), 52.

Higgins, B. (2005). Strategies for lowering attrition rates and raising NCLEX-RN pass rates. *Journal of Nursing Education, 44*(12), 541–547.

Hoffman, J. J. (2008). Teaching strategies to facilitate nursing students' critical thinking. *Annual Review of Nursing Education, 6,* 225–236.

Horns, P. N., O'Sullivan, P., & Goodman, R. (1991). The use of progressive indicators as predictors of NCLEX-RN success and performance of BSN graduates. *Journal of Nursing Education, 30,* 9–14.

Houltram, B. (1996). Entry age, entry mode and academic performance on a Project 2000 common foundation programme. *Journal of Advanced Nursing, 23*(6), 1089–1097.

Institute of Medicine (IOM). (2011). *The Future of Nursing: Leading Change: Advancing Health.* Washington, DC: The National Academies Press.

Kalisch, P. A., & Kalisch, B. J. (2004). American nursing: A history (4th ed.). Philadelphia, PA: Lippincott, Williams, & Wilkins.

Kelly, N. R., Shoemaker, M., & Steele, T. (1996). The experience of being a male student nurse. *Journal of Nursing Education, 29*(3), 118–121.

Kendall-Gallagher, D., Aiken, L. H., Sloane, D. M., & Cimotti, J. P. (2011). Nurse specialty certification, inpatient mortality, and failure to rescue. *Journal of Nursing Scholarship, 43*(2), 188–194.

Keogh, B. J., & O'Lynn, C. E. (2007). Gender-based barriers for male student nurses in general nursing education programs: An Irish perspective. In C. E. O'Lynn & R. E. Tranbarger (Eds.), *Men in Nursing: History, Challenges, and Opportunities* (pp. 193–204). New York, NY: Springer.

Kermode, S. (2006). Is nurse education sexist? An exploratory study. *Contemporary Nurse, 22*(1), 66–74.

Kevern, J., Rickett, C., & Webb, C. (1999). Pre-registration diploma students: a quantitative study of entry characteristics and course outcomes. *Journal of Advanced Nursing, 30*(4), 785–795.

Kvigne, K., & Kirkevold, M. (2002). A feminist perspective on stroke rehabilitation: The relevance of de Beauvoir's theory. *Nursing Philosophy, 3,* 79–89.

Lazarus, R. A., & Folkman, S. (1984). *Stress, appraisal, and coping.* New York: Springer.

Lecher, B. (2011). AAMN President's message to the membership. *InterAction, 29*(4), 22–26.

Le Hinds, N. (2010). *Male nurses: Gender-based barriers in nursing school.* Unpublished dissertation, Bernard School of Education, University of the Pacific, Stockton, CA.

Lewis, C., & Lewis, J. H. (2000). Predicting academic success of transfer nursing students. *Journal of Nursing Education, 39*(5), 188–192.

Lo, R., & Brown, R. (1999). Perceptions of nursing students on men entering nursing as a career. *Australian Journal of Advanced Nursing, 17*(2), 36–41.

Lou, J. H., Chen, S. H., Yu, H. Y., Li, R. H., Yang, C. I., & Eng, C. J. (2010). The influence of personality traits and social support on male nursing student life stress: A cross-sectional research design. *Journal of Nursing Research, 18*(2), 108–115.

Luhanga, F., Yonge, O. J., & Myrick. F. (2008). Failure to assign failing grades: Issues with grading the unsafe student. *International Journal of Nursing Education Scholarship, 5*(1), Article 8. **doi:** 10.2202/1548-923X.13661.

Luparell, S. (2004). Faculty encounters with uncivil nursing students: An overview. *Journal of Professional Nursing, 20*(1), 59–67.

Luparell, S. (2007). The effects of student incivility on nursing faculty. *Journal of Nursing Education, 46*(1), 15–19.

Luparell, S. (2011). Incivility in nursing: The connection between academia and clinical settings. *Critical Care Nurse, 31*(2), 92–95.

Magnussen, L. (2001). The use of cognitive behavior survey to assess nursing student learning. *Journal of Nursing Education, 40*(1), 43.

Malone, B., Tagliareni, E., Haney, K., Taylor, C., & Mancino, D. (2010). Your position in nursing: Realities of the current job market. *Imprint, 57*(3), 32–34.

Marchiondo, K., Marchiondo, L. A., & Lasiter, S. (2010). Faculty incivility: Effects on program satisfaction of BSN students. *Journal of Nursing Education, 49*(11), 608–614.

McDonald, P. J. (2010). Transitioning from clinical practice to nursing faculty: Lessons learned. *Journal of Nursing Education, 49*(3), 126–131.

McLaughlin, K., Muldoon, O. T., & Moutray, M. (2010). Gender, gender roles and completion of nursing education: A longitudinal study. *Nurse Education Today, 30*, 303–307.

McMillan, J., Morgan, S. A., & Arment, P. (2006). Acceptance of male registered nurses by female registered nurses. *Journal of Nursing Scholarship, 38*(1), 100–106.

McRae, M. J. (2003). Men in obstetrical nursing: Perceptions of the role. *MCN American Journal of Maternal-Child Nursing, 28*(3), 167–173.

Metz, A. M., Cech, E. A., Babcock, T., & Smith, J. L. (2011). Effects of formal and informal support structures on the motivation of Native American students in nursing. *Journal of Nursing Education, 50*(7), 388–394.

Milligan, F. (2001). The concept of care in male nurse work; on ontological hermeneutic study in acute hospitals. *Journal of Advanced Nursing, 35*(1), 7–16.

Moceri, J. T. (2010). Being cabezona: Success strategies of Hispanic nursing students. *International Journal of Nursing Education Scholarship, 7*(1), 1–15. doi: 10.2202/1548-923X.2036

Moscaritolo, L. M. (2009). Interventional strategies to decrease nursing student anxiety in the clinical learning environment. *Journal of Nursing Education, 48*(1), 17–23.

Mulholland, J., Anionwu, E. N., Atkins, R., Tappern, M., & Franks, P. J. (2008). Diversity, attrition and transition into nursing. *Journal of Advanced Nursing, 64*(1), 49–59.

National Council of State Boards of Nursing. (2011). *NCLEX examination pass rates.* Retrieved from http://www.ncsbn.org

National Council of State Boards of Nursing. (2012). *Computerized adaptive testing.* Retrieved from https://www.ncsbn.org/1216.htm

National League for Nursing. (2011a). *Retention rates in RN programs 2006–2007.* Retrieved from http://www.nln.org/research/slides/topic_retention_rn.htm

National League for Nursing. (2011b). *Certification for nurse educators.* Retrieved from http://www.nln.org/certification/index.htm

National League for Nursing. (2011c). *Re Health Affairs and the Nurse Educator Shortage.* Retrieved from http://www.nln.org/aboutnln/blast/blast_health_affairs_response.htm

National League for Nursing. (2011d). *Executive summary: Findings from the Annual Survey of Nursing Academic Year 2009–2010.* Retrieved from http://www.nln.org/research/slides/exec_summary_0910.pdf

Norman, L., Buerhaus, P. I., Donelan, K., McCloskey, B., & Dittus, R. (2005). Nursing students assess nursing education. *Journal of Professional Nursing, 21*(3), 150–158.

Nursing Standard. (2005). Students sink deeper in debt. *Nursing Standard, 19*(50), 14–17.

Okrainec, G. D. (1994). Perceptions of nursing education held by male nursing students. *Western Journal of Nursing Research, 16*(1), 94–107.

O'Lynn, C. (2003). *Defining male friendliness in nursing education programs. Tool development.* Unpublished dissertation, Kennedy-Western University, Cheyenne, WY.

O'Lynn, C. E. (2004). Gender-based barriers for male students in nursing education programs: Prevalence and perceived importance. *Journal of Nursing Education, 43*(5), 229–236.

Paterson, B. L., Tschikota, S., Crawford, M., Saydak, M., Venkatesh, P., & Aronowitz, T. (1996). Learning to care: Gender issues for male nursing students. *Canadian Journal of Nursing Research, 28*(1), 25–39.

Patterson, L., Grenny, J., McMillan, R., & Switzler, A. (2012). *Crucial conversations: Tools for talking when stakes are high* (2nd ed.). New York, NY: McGraw-Hill.

Plant, E. A., Ericsson, K. A., Hill, L., & Asberg, K. (2005). Why study time does not predict grade point average across college students: Implications of deliberate practice for academic performance. *Contemporary Educational Psychology, 30*, 96–116.

Pelican News. (2008). Financial aid for nursing education. Pelican News, 63(4), 12.

Potolsky, A., Cohen, J., & Saylor, C. (2003). Academic performance of nursing students: Do prerequisite grades and tutoring make a difference? *Nursing Education Perspectives, 24*(5), 246–250.

Popkess, A. M., & McDaniel, A. (2011). Are nursing students engaged in learning? A secondary analysis from the national survey of student engagement. *Nursing Education Perspectives, 32*(2), 89–94.

Pryjmachuk, S., Easton, K., & Littlewood, A. (2008). Nurse education: Factors associated with attrition. *Journal of Advanced Nursing, 65*(1), 149–160.

Purdue, G. L. (2009). Class preparation and study habits identified by associate degree nursing students. *Kentucky Nurse, 57*(2), 6.

Ramdass, D., & Zimmerman, B. J. (2011). Developing self-regulation skills: The important role of homework. *Journal of Advanced Academics, 22*(2), 194–218.

Rheaume, A. (2003). Establishing consensus about the baccalaureate entry-to-practice policy. *Journal of Nursing Education, 42*(12), 546–552.

Riddell, T. (2007). Critical assumptions: Thinking critically about critical thinking. *Journal of Nursing Education, 46*(3), 121–126.

Rossetti, J., & Fox, P. G. (2009). Factors related to successful teaching by outstanding professors: An interpretive study. *Journal of Nursing Education, 48*(1), 11–16.

Rouse, S. M., & Rooda, L. A. (2010). Factors for attrition in an accelerated baccalaureate nursing program. *Journal of Nursing Education, 49*(6), 359–361.

Ryan, S., & Porter, S. (1993). Men in nursing: A cautionary critique. *Nursing Outlook, 41*(6), 262–267.

Salamonson, Y., Andrew, S., & Everett, B. (2009). Academic engagement and disengagement as predictors of performance in pathophysiology among nursing students. *Contemporary Nurse, 32*(1–2), 123–132.

Salvage, J. (2000). The gender agenda. *Nursing Times, 96*(26), 26.

Sayles, S., & Shelton, D. (2005). Student success strategies. *The ABNF Journal. 16*(5), 98–101.

Simpson, R. (2005). Men in non-traditional occupations: Career entry, career orientation and experience of role strain. *Gender, Work, and Organization, 12*(4), 363–380.

Smith, J. S. (2006). Exploring the challenges for nontraditional male students transitioning into a nursing program. *Journal of Nursing Education, 45*(7), 263–269.

Sprouse, D. O. (1996). Message from the President. *InterAction, 14*(3)1–2, 4.

Spurlock, D. (2006). Do no harm: Progression policies and high-stakes testing in nursing education. *Journal of Nursing Education, 45*(8), 297–302.

Stott, A. (2007). Exploring factors affecting attrition of male students from an undergraduate nursing course: A qualitative study. *Nurse Education Today, 27*, 325–332.

Streubert, H. J. (1994). Male nursing students' perceptions of clinical experience. *Nurse Educator, 19*(5), 28–32.

Sullivan, E. J. (2000). Men in nursing: The importance of gender diversity. *Journal of Professional Nursing*, 16(5), 253–254.

Suplee, P. D., Lachman, V. D., Siebert, B., & Anselmi, K. K. (2008). Managing nursing student incivility in the classroom, clinical setting, and on-line. *Journal of Nursing Law*, *12*(2), 68–77.

Taylor, L. A., & Littleton-Kearney, M. (2011). Concept mapping: A distinctive educational approach to foster critical thinking. *Nurse Educator*, *36*(2), 84–88.

Tillman, K., & Machtmes, K. (2008). Masculinity. *Men in Nursing*, *3*(1), 23–28.

Timmons, F., & Kaliszer, M. (2002). Aspects of nurse education programmes that frequently cause stress to nursing students: fact finding sample survey. *Nurse Education Today*, 22, 203–211.

Urwin, S., Stanley, R., Jones, M., Gallagher, A., Wainwright, P., & Perkins, A. (2010). Understanding student nurse attrition: Learning from the literature. *Nurse Education Today*, 30, 202–207.

Watson, R., Gardiner, E., Hogston, R., Gibson, H., Stimpson, A., Wrate, R., & Deary, I. (2008). A longitudinal study of stress and psychological distress in nurses and nursing students. *Journal of Clinical Nursing*, 18, 270–278.

White, J., William, W. R., & Green, b. F. (1999). Discontinuation, leaving reasons and course evaluation comments of students on the common foundation programme. *Nurse Education Today*, 19, 142–150.

Wilgis, M., & McConnell, J. (2008). Concept mapping: An educational strategy to improve graduate nurses' critical thinking skills during a hospital orientation program. *Journal of Continuing Nursing Education*, *39*(3), 119–126.

Williams, C. L. (2001). The glass escalator: Hidden advantages for men in the "female" professions. In M. S. Kimmel & M. A. Messner (Eds.), *Men's lives* (5th ed., pp. 211–224). Needham Heights, MA: Allyn and Bacon.

Wilson, G. (2005). The experience of males entering nursing: A phenomenological analysis of professionally enhancing factors and barriers. *Contemporary Nurse*, *20*(2), 221–233.

Wittmann-Price, R. A., & Godshall, M. (Eds.) (2009). *Certified nurse educator (CNE) review manual*. New York: Springer

Wolkowitz, A. A., & Kelley, J. A. (2010). Academic predictors of success in a nursing program. *Journal of Nursing Education*, *49*(9), 498–503.

Wong, S. T., Seago, J. A., Keane, D., & Grumbach, K. (2008). College students' perceptions of their experiences: What to minority students think? *Journal of Nursing Education*, *47*(4), 190–195.

Wong, J., & Wong, S. (1999). Contribution of basic sciences to academic success in nursing education. *International Journal of Nursing Studies*, 36, 345–354.

US Department of Education. (2011). *Student aid eligibility.* Retrieved from http://studentaid.ed.gov/PORTALSWebApp/students/english/aideligibility.jsp

US Department of Education, Institute of Education Sciences. (2011). *Digest of education statistics: Table 331.* Retrieved from http://nces.ed.gov/programs/digest/d09/tables/dt09_331.asp

US Department of Education, Institute of Education Sciences. (2010). *Digest of education statistics*, 2009 (Chapter 3). (NCES 2010–013). Washington, DC: Author.

SIX

That's a Baby, Not a Football! Caring and Touch From a Man's Perspective

Although nursing has moved away from duty and womanly virtue as its main principles, caring has remained a central theme and core value in nursing (Chinn & Kramer, 2008). In fact, Clifford (1995) stated that there is no question that caring continues to be the center of nursing practice. Benner and Wrubel (1989) noted that caring is so important because caring is what matters to people, and caring is what people need in order to cope with the stress of illness. Many nurses believe that caring is what sets nursing apart from other health professions. So, it may be surprising that nurses have yet to define care and caring in clear and consistent terms. This problem continues probably because care and caring mean different things to different people and cultures (Leininger, 1991). I guess caring, like art, is in the eye of the beholder. In Western societies, caring has often been labeled as feminine and best suited for women. For the most part, men have accepted this label. Our Western society and dominant culture teaches men early in life that caring is not masculine. Boys are steered away from learning about caring and practicing caring on others. For example, boys often play with action figures instead of cuddly dolls; older boys mow lawns instead of babysit the neighbor's kids. Most boys grow up much more comfortable cradling a football than a baby.

I believe the feminine label given to caring is grossly inaccurate. This label has created enormous challenges for men in nursing. Conflicts arise when men, caring, and nursing are mixed together, which have fueled the historical discrimination against men in nursing and the continued barriers men in nursing still experience (see Chapters 2, 3, and 5). The reality is that men have cared for others throughout history and continue to do so today. The care men provide sometimes looks different from the care provided by women; but men's care is of value and is needed in nursing today. In this chapter, I will discuss care more deeply. I will offer a helpful description of caring, explain how caring became feminized, review what we know about how men care for others, and focus special attention on touch. My hope is that you will embrace and embody caring as a natural fit to your own maleness.

WHAT IS CARING?

Without a working definition of caring, it becomes difficult to determine what type of care is high-quality care and how nurses should provide care (Clifford, 1995; Morse, Solberg, Neander, Bottorff, & Johnson, 1990). Although authors don't agree on a definition of caring, most authors admit that care and caring are highly complex. Part of the complexity comes from the many ways the word *care* is used. Care may refer to an action, such as in caring for something or caring about something. In caring *for* something, a person acts to ensure the health and well-being of something or someone. In caring *about* something, a person has an emotional involvement, a passion, a love for the object he or she is caring for. Sometimes these phrases are used for separate things, such as "I care for my garden, and I care about students." Sometimes they are used for the same person, such as "I care for my elderly grandmother, and I care about her too." Care can mean a set of actions and behaviors, such as the care I receive from my nurse. And, caring can be used to describe someone, such as "my mother is a very caring person."

Capturing all the complexity of caring into a simple definition may be impossible. Paley (2001) complained that every new explanation of caring only repeats what has already been said on the topic, which doesn't lead to any clarity. I find his statements rather sour since he implied that we just leave the topic alone. But doing this would ignore the many studies that have shown the importance of caring; people can't stop caring about things, or caring for others. We must understand caring better, even if we can't define it, because caring matters to people.

I've read a number of articles, books, and theories about caring. Many of these have been written by nurses. One nurse theorist, Jean Watson, even founded an academic center devoted to understanding human caring. This center has brought scholars and clinicians together from around the world for over 25 years to study and learn about caring (University of Colorado College of Nursing, 2008). Many of these people have used this center and Watson's theories to explain caring. Others have used different theories. Of all that I read, I like the work of Janice Morse and her colleagues who published two articles about caring over 20 years ago (Morse, Solberg, Neander, Bottorff, & Johnson, 1990; Morse et al.,1991). These nurses examined the research on caring to date, synthesized the findings that were important for nurses, and created a model that identified the major components of caring and what caring by nurses should accomplish. Their work is clear, meaningful, and still current. It describes caring in a way that makes it easier to study and evaluate. Most important, their work illustrates that caring (and therefore nursing) is natural for all nurses, male *and* female.

Briefly, Morse et al. (1990, 1991) identified five interconnected perspectives of caring, all of which lead to two goals or outcomes. The five perspectives include:

- Caring as a human trait
- Caring as a moral imperative
- Caring as an affect

■ Caring as a nurse–patient relationship
■ Caring as a therapeutic intervention

The goals of these perspectives are a positive emotional (subjective) experience by the patient and a positive physical (objective) response by the patient. The assumption here is that effective care given by the nurse will achieve these goals of health and well-being. My only criticism of their work is that I feel there could be two other goals: positive emotional experience and physical response by the nurse. Effective care is not only good for the patient; it is also good for the nurse!

There is no order to the five perspectives; one is not more important than the other. They merely represent different ways of thinking about caring. *Caring as a human trait* suggests that all people can care. It is part of being human. That said, everyone has different skill levels for expressing care. Caring skill levels are influenced by our upbringing, our culture, and our experiences. *Caring as a moral imperative* means that caring is a value and an ideal for all nurses to strive for. As a value, caring drives all nursing actions. Since it is an ideal, we never give perfect care because humans aren't perfect. *Caring as an affect* means that in giving care, nurses create an empathetic feeling toward their patients. Caring implies a concern or interest in others and a dedication to the protection of others. *Caring as a nurse–patient relationship* means that the bond between the nurse and the patient is the spirit, or essence, of caring. This bond is visible to others. Actions that develop, strengthen, and maintain that bond define caring. And last, *caring as a therapeutic intervention* means that care is visible in all the actions nurses use to improve the patient's health. Nurses must have certain knowledge and skills in order to know when to use these actions in a way that is caring.

You may think that Morse et al. have only made the subject of caring more complicated. In some ways they have, since they gave us a fuller picture of care than have other authors. The reason I introduce you to their work in this chapter is to help you understand why labeling caring as feminine is inaccurate. All the perspectives of caring they present apply to both men *and* women. In the next sections, I discuss how caring became feminized and how men might display caring differently. As you read these sections, look back on these five perspectives. Hopefully, you will see that society has usually defined caring by using only bits and pieces of the five perspectives—bits and pieces that men and women might display differently, or bits and pieces that some people would label as feminine.

CARING: THE DOMAIN OF WOMEN?

According to James (1992), caring has been the responsibility of women in the family throughout time. Clearly, many people conjure up an image of a mother and child when they think about caring. That is not to say that men haven't cared for their families as well. Traditionally, however, men have left the home to obtain food and other resources for the family, or to protect the home and family from harm. These caring actions were just as necessary for the survival of the family as were the actions of women, who provided hands-on caring to children, the sick, and the elderly. Somewhere along the way, the caring actions of men were labeled differently. Even though the basic intent of men's and women's actions were the same (love of family and desire to ensure healthy survival of the family), their actions looked different and helped the family in different ways. Men's actions became known as *providing* for one's family instead of *caring* for one's family. It's quite possible that the need to separate the work of men from the work of women in patriarchal societies drove this distinction. The difference between men's and women's work came to be known as the *division of labor*. In patriarchal societies, men's work (providing) gained higher status and value than women's work (caregiving). This division in labor is the explanation used to support many of the beliefs, theories, and research about caring in our society, which has further cemented caring and caring behaviors in the domain of women (Stoller, 2002).

The family care provided by women usually happened in the privacy of the family home. Since caring was hidden in society and given low status, caring was ignored for centuries by scientists and researchers. Also, since caring happened in the home, caring was unpaid, which gave family care even lower status (James, 1992). Over the years, men offered various explanations to keep the status difference between women's work and men's work. It was explained that women did not have the intelligence, skill, or stamina for work beyond caregiving (see Chapter 3) or that it was women's duty (religious or otherwise) to care for the family and be subservient to men. Other explanations touted the virtues of women; that women were naturally good, loving, and charitable, which made them the best caregivers. These angelic qualities seem positive, but in reality, they proved to be a barrier for women. Since women were so virtuous and charitable, it was believed that women wouldn't ask or even want equal status and wages. After all, angels do not ask for money for their good works. Instead, it was believed that women's work should be done in the name of love. As I discussed in Chapter 3, these beliefs were also adopted by women, making these beliefs *societal* beliefs, not just the beliefs of men. As women moved into paid nursing roles outside the home, they were expected to provide caring as an extension of their family roles with minimum pay and self-sacrifice (Benner & Wrubel, 1989; James, 1992; Reversby, 1987). These beliefs about caring, and the consequences of these beliefs, have been the main target of feminist scholars over the years (Cancian & Oliker, 2000; Stoller, 2002; Thomas, 1993).

The image of the caring woman as the nurse was cemented in the public's mind by Nightingale herself, who noted that every woman was a nurse (2003/1859). As discussed in previous chapters, men were largely excluded from nursing schools from the time of Nightingale through the 1960s. As the number of male nurses dropped, the image of a caring woman (and not a man) as a nurse became a self-fulfilling prophecy. Lusk (2000) examined advertisements for nursing in hospital journals from 1930 to 1950 and noted that most were depicted as females who seemed eager to please the doctors and her patients. Takase, Kershaw, and Burt (2002) reviewed the research literature and noted that the public perception of nursing has been that nursing is a feminine occupation.

The connection between femininity and caring was boldly strengthened in academic circles by the work of Nancy Chodorow, who in the late 1970s wrote that women were more empathetic toward others because women have been influenced by their caregiving responsibilities in society (Stoller, 2002). On the other hand, society has influenced men to separate from emotional attachments and strive for self-independence. Also, Gilligan (1982) examined how men and women make decisions differently when faced with a moral conflict (see Chapter 5). Gilligan proposed that men tend to follow universal rules, an objective view of justice and what is right. Women tend to examine relationships and what matters to people. Women strive for a win-win outcome and use caring as the basis for their decisions—an approach Gilligan called an *ethic of care*. According to Tong (1993), Gilligan built on the work of Chodorow, believing that women show differences due to the societal and cultural messages about caring they receive their entire lives. Stoller (2002) suggested that these types of theories have been used to explain the research that finds men having different experiences of caring than women. This research creates a cycle where men are found to be different than women when providing care, and that caring is defined as feminine, further removing men from care. In other words, the divide between men and caring grows larger.

IS THERE A MASCULINE STYLE OF CARING?

This question is provocative. When I've asked this question of coworkers, I usually get puzzled looks. Some have told me, "No, everyone knows what caring is. Caring is caring." Others have said that men do caring differently than women, and that it's not as good as women's way of caring. In other words, there are masculine and feminine styles of caring, but they are not equal in value. Men's caring is compared to feminine standards, and it usually comes up short. This has also been the dominant belief of researchers for many years. Stoller (2002) stated that measuring men's caregiving with a "feminine yardstick" has become so common that it is barely noticed (p. 63). This belief creates a problem because it prevents us from understanding and learning from the ways men care for others (Stoller, 2002). It also becomes a problem because many men may not want to (or be able to) do caring in ways that women do caring.

The notion that men should somehow care like women is very challenging for men in nursing. Paterson, Crawford, Saydak, Venkatesh, Tschikota, and Aronowitz (1996) reported how uncomfortable male nursing students were with the expectations from female teachers that men care for their patients the way they [the teachers] did. I experienced this myself. As a student, I once cared for an elderly man who was very upset. My female teacher came in, held his hand, and talked in a soft, mother-like voice to him. The man seemed to feel better after this, but I knew I would never feel comfortable doing the same thing—taking an elderly man's hand into my own and talking to him in a maternal voice. At the time, I wondered if I would make a good nurse. Paterson et al. also reported that the male students learned on their own how to care in ways that they felt comfortable with as men. The same happened for me. I soon learned that I could touch an elderly man's shoulder for 10 seconds or so and give him words of encouragement, just as I would for a good friend. I realized that this approach would make him feel better, just like my teacher's hand-holding made him feel better.

Several studies have shown that men choose to become nurses because they want to care for and help others (Boughn, 2001; Hart, 2005; Ieradi, Fitzgerald, & Holland, 2010; Wilson, 2005), but the feminine yardstick is so common that even male nursing students believe they will have struggles trying to be as caring as their female classmates (Smith, 2006; Stott, 2007). Fortunately, male students can and do learn that they can demonstrate caring equally, although sometimes differently, than female students (Grady, Stewardson, & Hall, 2008; Paterson et al., 1996; Smith, 2006; Stott, 2007). But I worry about the self-doubt beginning male nursing students might have about their abilities, especially if these students face less-than-supportive female instructors (see Chapter 5). I believe that you will feel much better about your career choice if you understand more about caring and how men do caring.

So how do male nurses do caring differently than female nurses? The answer is unclear. Most of what we know about men's ways of caring has come from research on fathers and male family caregivers. In fact, a lot has been written on these types of caring by men, but this knowledge may not apply well to nursing. The relationship a father has with his child and the relationship a man has with an ill or disabled relative is very different from the relationship a male nurse has with his patient. Unfortunately, very little has been written about how male nurses differ from female nurses in their care. I think the family caregiver is closer to the role of nurse than that of a parent. A look at what we know about male family caregivers might be helpful.

In their ground-breaking book, Kramer and Thompson (2002) reviewed the research to date on male caregivers. Although there was much research, they noted that the quality of the research was often poor. They complained that even though men make up over 30% of all family caregivers, their experiences, and their contributions to society have largely been ignored. They reported that despite common myths, men experience some of the same stresses and health problems as do women when caring for a loved one at home. Thompson (2002) went on to say that because of major flaws in the research, there are many contradictions in the research findings. One important flaw has been that many researchers assume all men have the same beliefs, the same thoughts about masculinity, and make the same life choices.

Clearly, all men are different, but it cannot be denied that men are exposed to many of the same cultural and family messages about masculinity. Each man chooses to accept, revise, reprioritize, or reject the masculinity messages he encounters. I believe that the acceptance or rejection of a message may change over time or change upon the circumstances. For example, as a young man, you may think that men shouldn't be changing a baby's diaper. But as a husband and father, you may find it perfectly normal to change a baby's diaper. Or, as a boy, you may have thought that only girls grow up to be nurses. If there was a man who was a nurse, that wasn't normal. Now, you may have a very different idea about this particular masculinity message.

I believe how men respond to masculinity messages greatly influences how men do caring. If a man needs to care for others (e.g., a child or family member), or if a man chooses to care for others (e.g., nursing), he will need to resolve any conflicts caring work might have with masculinity messages. The process of resolving this conflict is called *negotiating gender*. In this process, the man has a conversation with himself, in which he has to negotiate which is more important: the caring work or the masculinity message. Sometimes, there is no noticeable negotiation. If he has already rejected a message, such as "men should not be nurses," then there is no conflict if he chooses to become a nurse. Since there is no conflict, there is nothing to negotiate. He pursues a nursing career and feels good about it. However, if caregiving (or some aspect of caregiving) does conflict with a masculinity message he has accepted, the internal negotiation begins. While this negotiation happens, the man may feel insecure, indecisive, anxious, or nervous. Earlier, I told you about my problem with caring for an elderly male patient by holding his hand. I wanted to make this patient more comfortable, but I had accepted the masculinity message that male strangers don't hold hands with emotion. This conflict caused me some anxiety because my teacher had not shown me other ways to demonstrate caring. Eventually, I negotiated a middle ground of sorts, by figuring out a way to touch and comfort him the same way I would touch and comfort a close friend. This resolved the conflict for me, and I still touch patients today in this same way.

Sometimes, the negotiation leads to a revision of the masculinity message. I found this play out in my own research (O'Lynn, 2010). I studied older men living in very rural areas in Montana and Oregon who were taking care of sick family members at home. After a number of interviews, I realized that these men had very little conflict about caregiving tasks. Most of them saw caregiving as work that had to be done; caregiving wasn't manly work or womanly work. Caregiving was a job that anyone should do if needed. Some of the men saw caregiving as a family obligation. Others saw caregiving as something you did out of love for your family. But caregiving is hard work, often with responsibilities 24 hours a day/7 days a week. These men needed help, or at least a daily break. All these men had grown up with the masculinity message that men should be self-sufficient; men don't ask for help for work that could be done on their own. This created a conflict. Some of the men clung on to that masculinity message; they never asked for help. They insisted that they could do it on their own. These men were stressed out. They were neglecting their caregiving, which put their sick family member at risk of harm. These men couldn't get other work done. These men reported having stress-related health problems of their own, including symptoms of depression. Some of them resorted to alcohol to escape the stress. In short, their firm acceptance of this masculinity message was making them sick, miserable, and poor caregivers.

Some of the men rejected the masculinity message of not asking for help, so they had no conflict. They asked for help right away. Still other men revised their masculinity messages. When they first became caregivers, they experienced some of the same turmoil as the first group of men. For some of them, things got so bad that they had to swallow their pride and ask for help.

For others, neighbors stepped in and insisted on helping out and wouldn't take "no" for an answer! The men saw the benefit of the help they were getting, and soon asked for more help when necessary. Soon, they were feeling better, were getting other work done, and their family members were getting better care. These men didn't reject the masculinity message completely; they still did everything they could by themselves. But these men allowed themselves to ask for help when things got tough. In other words, they revised the message to include exceptions. Going back to my earlier example of holding the hand of an elderly male patient, I still don't offer my hand to elderly male patients normally. However, if the *patient* reaches for my hand to hold, I don't turn him away. In other words, I have revised my own masculinity message to include the exception of the patient taking *my* hand first.

Perhaps the most interesting form of negotiation is the one of reprioritizing multiple masculinity messages. One man I interviewed told me that he also accepted the message of not asking for help. On the other hand, this man also accepted the masculinity message of being a good provider: that a man should take care of his family. Initially, he resisted asking for help with his caregiving work. As he started to wear down, he could see how his family member was suffering from his poor caregiving. At this point, he realized that he was not taking good care of his family, so he asked for help. In other words, the good provider message was more important than the self-sufficiency message. As things at home improved, he didn't see himself as someone who couldn't do things on his own. Instead, he saw himself as a better provider for his family.

Revising and reprioritizing masculinity messages have been reported by other researchers. Wall (2009) noticed that men belonging to the Alexian Brothers (a Catholic order for men) see their nursing and service work not as feminine, but as a display of their spirituality, faith, and religious obligation. Similarly, Solari (2006) interviewed Russian Orthodox Christian immigrant men working as home caregivers in San Francisco. These men did not see their work as womanly, but rather as charitable and spiritual. Solari further noted that men who revised or reprioritized messages were much happier and more engaged in their work than either men or women who viewed their caregiving as paid employment.

I believe the negotiation of masculinity messages leads to the differences in caring you might see between men and women. Negotiation is unique to men in this area of caring, since women don't have to negotiate femininity messages in order to care for others (though they may have to negotiate family role messages, relationship messages, or other types of messages as they enter the workforce as nurses). Thompson (2002) noted that there are some common ideas from the research about how men do caring differently than women. According to Thompson's review, men readily step up to the plate when needed to care for family members, though husbands tend to spend more time caring for their wives and are more likely to perform personal care than are sons toward a parent. Husbands tend to look at caregiving as an extension of their marriage vows. They enjoy the challenge of caregiving and seek information to solve specific caregiver problems. They are often stoic, not seeking help from homecare services, and readily give up old routines so that they can take on new duties, such as housework. On the other hand, sons are more likely to have jobs and other family obligations. They are more likely to use the assistance of others and hire homecare services when available (Thompson, 2002).

The research suggests that many men use what's called a professional model when caring for family members (Thompson, 2002). In this model, men view their caregiving activities as work, similar to a job. They adopt a managerial style to their caregiving. Men focus on tasks that need to be completed. They do not let the caregiving work consume them emotionally or spirituality. Men are more likely than women to keep outside interests and maintain social relationships with other family members and friends. Men are more likely to separate caregiving from the other things in their lives. In other words, caregiving responsibilities are a *part* of their lives, but do not take over their lives. Some have called this caregiving approach cold and uncaring, but men who use this approach report that they include nurturing into their caregiving work. Men report deeper intimacy and emotional ties with their loved ones as a result of their caregiving work.

Like women, men are at risk for stress, depression, and emotional and physical exhaustion from caregiving. However, since they keep outside interests and relationships alive, men seem to suffer the consequences of caregiving less than women. This ability is actually a benefit which may make men able to endure lengthy caregiving in a more healthy fashion (Thompson, 2002). I saw much of this in my own research. The happiest caregivers were those that were able to keep outside interests and stay connected with others. They took breaks during the day, and took days off in order to re-energize themselves. Most of the men talked about and approached caregiving as if it was a job, but they also talked about the deep emotional connection they had with their family members. They had a sense of pride in their caregiving and the deeper relationships that had developed with their loved ones (O'Lynn, 2010).

Unlike the research on male caregivers and fathers, there is almost no research on how male nurses care for their patients. A Canadian study completed in the 1990s resulted in two articles (Paterson, Tschikota, Crawford, Saydak, Venkatesh, & Aronowitz, 1995;, Paterson et al., 1996). In the first article, Paterson et al. described how male nursing students learned how to care. The men reported that they believed caring was a trait everyone possessed in varying degrees. They believed that their clinical experiences built and refined their abilities to care for others. Beginning students reported that they learned much from seeing behaviors that were negative and not caring. These uncaring behaviors included gossiping, being judgmental, focusing only on tasks and not the emotional component of care, and doing the minimum amount of work possible. In research circles, this type of observation is called a negative case. Much can be learned from seeing what *not* to do, but students also reported learning much from seeing examples of good caring, mostly from the other nurses and their classmates. Both junior and senior students saw these nurses as role models. In addition, senior students reported learning how to care by hearing and reflecting on the stories told to them by patients and experienced nurses. From these stories, students were able to connect past experiences with new experiences. The students were better able to understand the complicated picture of patient care (Paterson et al., 1995).

In their second article, Paterson et al. (1996) focused on the differences the male students saw in themselves compared to their female teachers and classmates. The researchers reported that observing the gender differences, living through the differences, and preparing themselves for the differences all led to the men's ability to learn "caring as a male" (p. 29). Junior students noticed that women were very open about showing feelings of love, sensitivity, and caring toward their patients. The men noted that the women were very touchy-feely. The men were frustrated because they could see the positive effects of touchy-feely care, but these actions went against what they were taught about masculinity. One student said, "I feel like if I acted the way my teachers wanted me to, with all that touchy-feely stuff, that I'd have to become less of a man. I'd have to act like a woman, not a man" (p. 30). The students also felt that their teachers didn't understand this conflict, or possibly, didn't care that the students were frustrated. The senior students, however, had learned how to incorporate the styles of all nurses into a hybrid style of caring. Sometimes, this happened by watching a male nurse. The students reported that a masculine style of caring was less touchy-feely, and more of a friendship. One student said this:

> I was amazed at the relationship he [male nurse] had with his patients. He was loud at times. He told jokes. He teased them a lot. But they loved him. And you could tell he cared about them deeply. I think some of the female nurses on the unit thought he was too casual and not caring enough. I think they were wrong. (p. 32)

By observing this male nurse, the male students were able to see a style of caring that was more compatible with their own masculinities. Another student commented, "I would just like to talk to some [male nurses] and hear about their experiences. I think they could teach me more about being a male in nursing than my female teachers can" (p. 34).

Paterson et al.'s (1996) suggestion that senior students develop a hybrid style is similar to my earlier discussion on gender negotiation. The male students observed caring behaviors from both women and men. They understood that blending the two would result in an honest caring style without unacceptable conflicts with masculinity. These men negotiated a style that would make them effective nurses, even though that style might differ somewhat from women. The development of a hybrid style through negotiation was also implied in a study by Tillman and Machtmes (2008). These researchers interviewed eight men in the southern United States. These men felt that being empathetic and caring was not a conflict with masculinity. In school, they learned how to communicate in a more caring manner and listen better to patients' needs. Displaying more caring communication did not make them feel less like men.

The idea of different styles of caring and the possibility that different styles might be a strength of diversity have not been discussed much by authors. In fact, most nurses learned that there is only one right way to do things, including caring. However, the topic of different styles of care is not completely absent from nursing articles. Morse et al. (1990) reported that nurses don't care for patients all in the same way. Nurses show different styles of interactions with patients depending upon the clinical situation. They said:

> To the patient who is perceived to be suffering, the nurse's tone may be quiet and empathetic; to the confused patient, directive or persuasive; to the patient experiencing pain, encouraging; and so forth. Moreover, to the depressed patient who is beginning to respond, the nurse may be teasing, or to the young orthopedic patient, the nurse may be authoritarian. (p. 10)

Morse et al. stated that more research is needed about different caring styles. Some 22 years later, I have not found much more information about caring styles, who is more likely to use which style, and which style might be better to use in certain situations. The research has been rather vague. For example, Milligan (2001) interviewed eight male nurses in England. These men described what they felt was important in caring. The men reported that the only differences they saw in their caring compared to their female coworkers is that the women were more likely to show emotions, such as crying when a patient dies. The men also reported that they were aware that they were in a minority status, and that not all patients are as comfortable with men as their nurses. Milligan worried about men not receiving the emotional support and encouragement from other nurses that they might need. Dahlberg (1994) noted that in Sweden, women are better than men in seeing patients as a whole person. Women seek intimacy and connection with others, making them better caregivers and nurses. Men seek power and control. Dahlberg suggested that other health care fields dominated by men (e.g., medicine, administration) should teach their students the way nurses are taught! Gilloran (1995) interviewed 15 nurses working on a psychiatry unit in Scotland. The male nurses reported that they were more confident in their decision-making ability than the female nurses, and that men were less touchy feely and more rational and academic in their approach with patients. The female nurses reported that men were lazier, paid less attention to detail, and were more interested in promotions than were the female nurses. Interestingly, none of these nurses discussed positive contributions made by nurses of the opposite sex. It's possible that this unit was overshadowed by poor working relations and negativity. Grady et al. (2008) interviewed teachers at a nursing school. Overall, the teachers didn't see much difference between male and female students. They recognized that men come to nursing as caring persons and that their caring skills are further developed in nursing school. Some of the teachers said that the men *felt* that it took them longer to reach their potential than female students, but that all the men demonstrated caring. Another teacher emphasized that any differences in caring among students was due to individual factors more than gender. However, one of the teachers interviewed was male. He reported that the men needed male teachers because male teachers, "…are better able to identify and appreciate male nursing students' expressions of caring" (p. 318). This male teacher said further that men don't display their caring always the same was as women, but that the caring is of equal value to the caring done by women. He said he encourages male students to reflect on which types of caring are important and feel comfortable to each student. These studies only touch the surface of caring styles.

Based on what I have read, and based on my experiences and those told to me by other men, I believe that men come to nursing with the ability to care and the desire to care. Men place value on caring. In their roles as nurses, men want to use various actions to improve the patient's comfort and well-being. Any differences in caring between men and women, I believe, happen in how that care is displayed and the nature of the relationships male nurses develop with their patients. Masculinity messages influence how men display caring. Some men reject some of these messages. Most male nurses revise or reprioritize the messages to create a caring style that is all their own. (By the way, I believe some female nurses have to negotiate femininity messages as well. For example, nurses need to confront others when a situation might harm a patient. Confronting others may pose conflict with a femininity message, and therefore, must be negotiated.) If a man has trouble negotiating conflicts with multiple masculinity messages, he may leave nursing, or he may not have pursued a nursing career in the first place.

Probably, it is not all that important to try to understand feminine styles of caring and masculine styles of caring per se. I fear that such work might imply that men should always use a masculine style and that women should always use a feminine style. Instead, it is more important that you understand the idea of negotiating masculinity messages so that you may develop your own style of caring that feels right for you and meets the patient's needs. After all, what is most important is improving the patient's comfort and well-being. In my mind, that is far more important than how the caring looks.

That said, there is one masculinity message that is especially difficult for men to negotiate: touch. In my own research, men reported that their struggles with touch created one of the most difficult barriers for them in school (Keogh & O'Lynn, 2007; Le-Hinds, 2010; O'Lynn, 2004). I have seen this struggle with my own male students. Since conflicts with touch are so important, the next section will be devoted to touch and how to reduce any conflicts you might have about providing touch as a nurse.

WORRIES OVER TOUCH: A BARRIER TO CARING

There are many ways to show caring to patients, but no other caring activity in nursing has received as much attention as has touch. In fact, multiple authors have said that touch is an essential way that nurses communicate caring to their patients (Estabrooks, 1987; Evans, 2002; Kidd & Wagner, 2001; Kozier, Erb, Berman, & Snyder, 2004; Leininger, 1991; Riley, 2004). Yet men report touch as one of the most important conflicts they have with masculinity messages. Evans stated further that men's touch has become highly sexualized in today's society. Men's fears that patients will interpret their touch as having a sexual nature or intent, whether or not the patient is male or female, has been reported in multiple studies, including my own research (Edwards, 1998; Evans, 2002; Gleeson & Higgins, 2009; Harding, North, & Perkins, 2008; Inoue, Chapman, & Wynaden, 2006; Keogh & Gleeson, 2006; Keogh & O'Lynn, 2007; O'Lynn, 2004).

What's interesting to me is that even though touch is such an important caring yet fearful activity, exactly how and when to touch patients are hardly discussed at all in nursing school. I examined seven basic nursing textbooks commonly used in the United States and found almost no instructions on touch, and no specific instructions for men (O'Lynn, 2007). Nurses reported that they didn't learn how to touch patients in nursing school, but figured it out on their own based on their past experiences before becoming a nurse or by trial-and-error once they have become nurses (Estabrooks & Morse, 1992; Keogh & Gleeson, 2006; Paterson et al., 1996). Nurses also reported that they are frustrated that they had to figure out how to touch patients on their own (Paterson et al., 1996; Van Dongen & Elema, 2001).

In my experience, all students have questions about touch when they start nursing school. Female students, however, tend to have different questions than male students. I have found that women often worry that male patients will think that the female nurse is flirting, or coming on to him if she touches him in a certain way. Men worry about this too, but usually only if the patient is another male. If the patient is a woman, men often worry that she might think he is sexually assaulting her. I believe teachers need to talk to students about these concerns right away, at the very beginning of the nursing coursework. Without this discussion, some men's worries might escalate, creating a significant barrier for their learning and development of nursing skills.

Several years ago, a colleague and I developed a special touch class and lab, and offered it to students. We learned that it was better to separate the men and women in this class. Many men, and some women, were nervous about asking certain questions in a mixed class. Separating the students created discussions that were more in-depth and honest. In this class and lab, we show exactly how, when, and where to touch patients. The techniques we teach help reduce students' anxieties about touch, and help students ensure that their touch is interpreted as professional and displays dignity. I'd like to share these techniques with you.

Purpose of Touch

Much is written about touch, but before 1990, most of the published articles focused on defining touch and explaining its purposes (Routasalo, 1999). Estabrooks (1989) described the types of touch used in nursing. She noted three types of touch: instrumental touch, expressive touch, and protective touch. The first type, instrumental, is touch required to complete a task. For example, if you are going to take a patient's blood pressure, you have to touch the patient's arm to place the blood pressure cuff. The purpose of this touch is to complete a task, nothing more. Because this touch is required to complete a task, it has also been called "necessary touch." The second type, expressive, is touch given to a patient in order to provide comfort or emotional support. An example might be holding someone's hand who is upset, or patting someone on the back to offer congratulations. This type of touch has also been called "comforting touch," "nonprocedural touch," or "unnecessary touch" because this touch is voluntary on the part of the nurse. The third type, protective, is touch used to prevent the patient from injury. For example, the nurse might push the hand of a confused patient away from a piece of dangerous equipment. A single touch encounter may have more than one purpose. Let's say you are taking care of a gentleman whose balance is very poor. You are helping him stand up and walk by holding on to his arm and waist. You could think of this touch as being of all three types: instrumental, in that you have to hold on to him to give him balance; expressive, in that your grip on the patient will help lower his anxiety about standing up; and protective, in that your touch will help prevent him from falling and hurting himself.

Since the 1990s, most of the articles on touch have focused on how often nurses use different types of touch. Most studies have shown that instrumental touch is used far more often than expressive touch, and that nurses and patients are usually comfortable with instrumental touch (Edwards, 1998; Gleeson & Timmons, 2005; McCann & McKenna, 1993; Routasalo & Isola, 1996; Williams, 2001). When expressive touch is used, nurses usually touch patients' arms, hands, shoulders, and knees. Many patients find this type of touch comfortable, but some patients don't, depending upon the situation (Gleeson & Timmons, 2005; Fisher & Joseph, 1989; Hollinger & Buschmann, 1993; McCann & McKenna, 1993; Mulaik et al., 1991; Routasalo & Isola, 1996). I have not found much written about protective touch. I believe some authors consider protective touch a type of instrumental touch.

Intimate Touch

One type of instrumental touch seems to be the core of most people's anxieties about touch: a type of touch called *intimate touch*. I define intimate touch as touch to areas of the body that might produce feelings of unease, anxiety, or fear, or are likely to be misinterpreted as sexual in nature. Unease with intimate touch can be felt by the nurse, the patient or both. Although each person is different, the parts of the body related to intimate touch include the genitals, crotch area, buttocks, inner thighs, lower abdomen, and the breasts. Intimate touch is *always* instrumental touch. You should never touch these body parts for emotional or comforting purposes. Touch to these areas is used only to accomplish a task, such as listening to the heart with your stethoscope or giving someone a bath who can't do it themselves. Intimate touch is used frequently in nursing. Unfortunately, intimate touch can create negative feelings from the patient even if the nurse has very good intentions.

I noticed the struggles my male students had with intimate touch. My students understood they had to touch their patients' bodies. They wanted to know the nuts-and-bolts of how to do the touch. I looked for research that might help me teach the students to develop good touch skills, but I found very little. What I did find only mentioned that intimate touch made men nervous. I already knew that. I found nothing specific on how to provide intimate touch. For example, where do you place your hands on the body? When do you place your hands on the body? How should you touch? Firmly? Gently?

I took what little information I could find and added my own thoughts based on my experiences as a nurse. I asked other nurses for their suggestions, and eventually, came up with a list of intimate touch techniques. I taught these techniques in a class and lab and asked the students whether they thought the techniques were helpful. I made a few changes. Then, I presented the information at a national conference. Those at the conference gave me a few more suggestions. I made some more changes. By this time, I teamed up with a coworker, Lorretta Krautscheid. Lorretta told me that she also noticed that students struggle with intimate touch. I told her about the techniques. She thought they made a lot of sense, and suggested that we offer a touch lab to all the students. We taught the touch lab to a group of students and got their feedback for any more changes. Lorretta and I thought it would be a good idea to go back to the research and see if there was any new information. We didn't find much, but what surprised us most was that all the articles were based only on the opinions of nurses. In other words, we couldn't find anything where *patients* were asked how *they* thought nurses should provide intimate touch. So, Lorretta and I got several groups of people together and asked them about intimate touch. We were relieved that people said pretty much what we had already put together (O'Lynn & Krautscheid, 2011). After all the input from students, teachers, nurses, and the general public, I am confident that the following intimate touch principles are on target.

Innocent until proven guilty

This first principle is probably the most important and obvious principle. You need to remember that you are a professional and have good moral and ethical intentions. You need to understand why you are touching your patient and determine whether or not touch is necessary. You need to be confident that the patient will trust you. Believing in yourself is necessary if you are going to project professionalism. When you project professionalism, others are more likely to assume that your intentions are good, and that you will use intimate touch appropriately.

No automatic chaperones and no use of the word "chaperone"

Policies that require men to have a chaperone for tasks that involve intimate touch are degrading. These policies negate the male nurse's presumed innocence and good intentions. The automatic use of chaperones creates a lose-lose situation, in which trust is damaged. The assumed purpose of a chaperone is either to protect the patient from a nurse who might do something inappropriate (the nurse cannot be trusted); or the chaperone is to protect the nurse from false accusations from the patient (the patient cannot be trusted); or both. A policy that requires automatic chaperones assumes the worst of people. The only person that should decide whether or not a chaperone is necessary should be the *patient*. The patient's comfort is what is important here. Some patients may prefer a chaperone; others are modest and would prefer to have as few people involved with an intimate procedure as possible. Asking the patient directly whether or not a chaperone is needed has become the expectation and standard in the United Kingdom (Nursing and Midwifery Council, 2008).

If the patient requests a chaperone, who you chose for this job is very important. In many situations, you will want another nurse or a nurse's aide, since these persons could assist you with the task that requires intimate touch. In other words, getting a secretary to chaperone while you insert a catheter (tube) into a patient's bladder would not be ideal. The secretary isn't trained in how to do this task. The secretary will only be able to stand and watch. This might make the patient feel uncomfortable. A person who only stands and watches a procedure could seem like a witness to a potential crime. This type of a chaperone can further erode any trust between the nurse and the patient. In some situations, such as working with small children, you may want to have a parent or guardian assist you. Using parents can be tricky when working with teenagers, so check with your charge nurse or teacher in these situations. Sometimes, an adult may want his or her spouse to be a chaperone.

The second part of this principle is to *not* use the word chaperone when speaking with patients. We found that people have very negative images of the word chaperone, making them think of parents having to chaperone teenagers because they fear teenagers won't behave appropriately (O'Lynn & Krautscheid, 2011). Instead, when talking with patients, use the words *helper* or *assistant*. These words are more positive and imply that the other person will be actively helping instead of just standing in the room watching.

Building rapport

Rapport is a connection, a relationship with another. Rapport must be established before intimate touch happens. Rapport doesn't require a large amount of time; rapport can be created quickly by giving patients your full attention and listening to their needs. In terms of intimate touch, you must communicate with your patients. Whenever possible, let patients know that you will need to touch them. If it is not obvious, explain where you will touch them and why you will need to touch them *before* you physically touch their bodies. This was one of the most important things people told us in our study; they want their nurses to tell them what they plan on doing before they do it (O'Lynn & Krautscheid, 2011).

Building rapport is easier when you project a professional image. What you have heard about making a good first impression applies here. Make sure you are dressed appropriately and follow your employer's dress code. Stand up straight and keep good posture. Do not address your patients in a manner that is too casual, unless the patient prefers that. Don't speak to your adult patients in a child-like manner. Make sure you use good grammar, avoid slang, and never use foul language. Listen to your patients. Observe their body gestures and positions for clues on how they are feeling. When you project a professional image, you are more likely to earn the patient's respect. This will make it easier to build rapport and gain the patient's trust.

Another way to build rapport is to reduce power differentials. Patients often feel vulnerable. They are sick and have to rely on other people to do things for them. Sometimes, they have to rely on others to help them with very personal tasks, such as using the restroom. For some patients, this makes them feel that the nurse has a lot of power over them. One way to reduce this power difference is to position yourself eye-to-eye with your patients when you need to talk to them about intimate touch. Standing over a patient creates a position of power. When you sit or squat down so you can be at the eye level of the patient, you create a position of equality.

Another way to reduce power is to offer patients choices about intimate touch. People told us that they wanted to decide whether or not intimate touch was necessary, and if it was, they wanted to determine how intimate touch was going to occur. Allow patients to do as much personal care as they can, then offer your help to do what they cannot do. Don't just automatically do things for the patient. As you offer choices, also seek permission from the patient to do the task that will require intimate touch. The patient may be OK with you doing the task, or the patient may want to do it themselves (if they are able), or have another person do the task instead of you. If the patient wants someone else to do the task, don't be offended. The patient's preference may have nothing to do with you personally; they just may be more comfortable having someone else help with a private task. Remember, nursing care is *not* about you, it's about the patient. The patient's preferences need to be respected. Soon, I'll give an example of how rapport building might work.

Ensuring privacy

Whenever you provide intimate touch, make sure the setting is as private as possible. Close the door, pull the curtains, or draw the blinds to prevent others outside the room from seeing the patient's body. Also, expose the patient's body as minimally as possible. This may seem like common sense, but it is amazing how often nurses forget to do this. Sometimes, the nurse doesn't realize that the patient feels that there is a loss of privacy. For example, one person told us about using the bathroom in her hospital room. She resented how her nurse would leave the bathroom door open when the patient was using it. Other nurses would stand in the bathroom while she was taking a shower. I assume the nurses did this to see if the patient was able to do her hygiene safely, but the patient didn't know this. If you need to supervise the patient, explain this to the patient, and help the patient with the activity. If you want to see if the patient can do everything independently, then give the patient encouragement and support. In other words, don't just passively watch the patient. As this patient told us, "Don't just stand there and watch me bathe. Help, or get out!" (O'Lynn & Krautscheid, 2011, p. 29).

Just right with touch

When you start the touch, touch the patient with confidence. Shaking hands will show the patient that you are uncomfortable. If you look uncomfortable, the patient will be more anxious. Several people told us how important it was that the touch feels just right. They didn't want touch that was too gentle, or touch that was too rough. They didn't want the nurse to go too fast with intimate touch; this gave the message that the nurse was uncomfortable and just wanted to get the task over with. This felt impersonal to the patient, as if they weren't human. On the other hand, people told us that they didn't want the touch to be too slow; this made the touch seem lingering and creepy (O'Lynn & Krautscheid, 2011). The way to get the touch just right is to pay attention to the patient while you are touching them. Some patients will tell you right away if your touch is uncomfortable, but if the patient is nervous with your touch, often they will not say anything. Instead, patients may show their discomfort nonverbally. Watch the patient's facial expressions and body language when you use intimate touch. If they appear uncomfortable, then stop. Ask them if they are OK. Get feedback from the patient so you will be better at getting the touch just right. And remember, just right for *this* patient may not be just right for the *next* patient, or for the same patient but at a different time. This means that you must pay attention to the patient *every* time you use intimate touch.

Progressive touch
This principle speaks to the sequence of your touch. If at all possible, the first contact you make with a patient's body should *not* be the most sensitive part of their body. For example, if you need to wash someone who has messed the bed, don't start by cleaning the genitals. Wash another body part first. Or, if you need to lift up a woman's breast so you can listen to her heart with your stethoscope, start by listening to a different part of the chest, and then move her breast. In other words, touch safer parts of the body before touching more sensitive body parts. This will allow the patient a little time to get used to the feeling of your hand on his or her body.

Distraction
The purpose of distraction is to help patients get their minds off of thinking about your hand on their bodies. You can distract patients two ways: engage them in meaningful conversation and use concurrent touch. When you are using intimate touch, avoid silence while touching. Silence allows patients to become more anxious. Instead, fill the silence with meaningful conversation. Don't use this time to air complaints, gossip, or chatter on about your own interests and personal life. Instead, use this time to ask the patient questions, explain things, or make polite small talk. If your conversation makes the patient think about answering your questions, their minds will more easily drift away from the intimate touch. Also, distract patients by using concurrent touch. Concurrent touch occurs when you touch two different parts of the body at the same time, the sensitive body part and a body part that is less sensitive. Concurrent touch distracts the brain. Patients won't be as focused on the sensation of your hand touching only sensitive areas. This takes a bit of practice, but this skill will become natural for you in a short period of time. Concurrent touch doesn't only involve the hands. You can touch people with other parts of your body. For example, when cleaning the genitals, your hands may be busy cleaning, but you can touch the patient's knee with your forearm or elbow. This is also helpful if you need to keep your hands sterile. When listening to the chest, your hand holding the stethoscope may be

touching a woman's breast, but your other hand could be gently resting on her shoulder.

Cultural considerations

The last principle pertains to culture. Some cultures do not allow members of the opposite sex to use intimate touch on people who are not immediate family members. This may prevent you from using intimate touch on some patients. Be sensitive to this, and respect the cultural customs of patients.

Intimate touch example

Let's look at an example of how these principles might be used. Let's say I am taking care of Mrs. Johnson, an elderly woman who had surgery on her hip. She can move around the bed a little, but she's not allowed to get out of bed yet. This morning, she used a bedpan, but tipped it over after using it. Now she and her bed are wet with urine. She will need to be washed up and have her bed sheets changed. Let's say I'm just starting my day. I haven't met Mrs. Johnson yet. My conversation with her might go something like this:

"Hello Mrs. Johnson. My name is Chad O'Lynn. I am your nurse today. I heard you had an accident in your bed. I'm sorry about that.... Is it OK if I help you get cleaned up?"

Mrs. Johnson nods her head and says, "Yes, that would be fine."

"May I take a quick look under the covers to see what I need to get?" I ask.

Mrs. Johnson looks away, frowns, and nods her head. She doesn't say anything.

"What's wrong Mrs. Johnson? Is there anything I can do?"

"This is all so embarrassing. And I've never had a man do something like this for me."

I sit down on a chair next to her bed so that I am closer to her eye level. "I hear you," I tell her. "If it's any consolation, I've cleaned up a lot of messes. I will be very respectful, but if you would like, I can have Sally come in and help me."

Mrs. Johnson looks at me and shakes her head. "No, that's okay. Let's just get this finished with."

I get up and shut the door. I lift her covers partially and see that I only need to change her pad and the pillow case on the pillow by her feet. I gather my supplies and raise her bed up to a good working level. I give her a warm soapy washcloth and ask if she would like to clean herself up below.

"No, I can't. That's the problem, otherwise, I would do it myself," she tells me.

"That's okay. I'll take care of it, but first I'll get your leg and foot cleaned up." I place some towels under her leg and wash her foot and lower leg, then work upward toward her upper leg and crotch area. I watch her facial expressions for any signs of discomfort. She looks okay. "Has the doctor been in to see you yet this morning?" I ask her.

"No. I haven't seen him yet, but the physical therapist came in and told me that she was going to get me in a chair this morning if it's okay with the doctor. I'm a little nervous about that," Mrs. Johnson says.

I begin to tell Mrs. Johnson how it works the first time a patient gets out of bed. I go over some safety precautions. I tell her that I can give her some medication so that she won't be in too much pain. I ask her several questions about pain medications and which ones worked well for her in the past. Meanwhile, I keep washing. As I begin to wash her sensitive areas, I have my right elbow resting very gently on her knee. I keep watching her facial expressions. She looks okay. I ask her to turn on her side so I can wash her buttocks. I help her on her side and support her hip with my hand. I clean her with the washcloth in my other hand. When I am done, I pat her dry and place a clean pad under her. When I'm finished, I remove my gloves and straighten out her blankets. "Was that okay?" I ask her.

Mrs. Johnson looks at me and smiles, "Yes, that was fine."

"Great," I say. I place my hand gently on her shoulder. "I'll get this room cleaned up for you before breakfast gets here." I get everything straightened up. Before I leave, I tell her that I will make sure she has her pain medications before she has therapy. As I open the door, I turn around and give her a smile. "I'm here for you Mrs. Johnson. All you have to do is call."

SUMMARY

Over the years, caring has been labeled as feminine and women's work by theorists, scholars, and by the general public. This label has been inaccurate since men have cared for others as far back as we know, and continue to care for others today. Researchers and authors have done little to clarify caring or recognize the value of the caring provided by men. Instead, researchers and authors have focused on the differences between how men and women experience caregiving. Furthermore, many researchers and scholars use the way women do caring as the gold standard. If men do caring differently than women, then by definition, men's caring is not as true, not as good as women's caring. Morse, Solberg, S. M., Neander, W. L., Bottorff, J. L., & Johnson (1990) provided a model to look at caring more fully. From their model and from the research presented in this chapter, men have the ability and desire for caring, and men place value on caring. Generally, differences between men's and women's caring come in the way the caring is displayed, but these differences do not get in the way of meeting the goals for caring. I believe differences in men's caring happen due to the need to negotiate any conflicts between caring and the masculinity messages men receive from family, peers, and society. Since caring has been perceived as women's work, women do not experience the conflicts with caring that men do, and therefore, have little need for negotiating caring with femininity messages.

One important activity in caring, touch, creates important conflicts for many men for two reasons. First, touch is a common way women display caring. How often, the way, and where women touch others conflicts with masculinity messages for many men; yet male nursing students have reported that they are taught to use feminine ways of touching. Second, men's touch has been sexualized in our society. Increasing media attention on sexual assaults by men has promoted the belief that men's touch should be viewed suspiciously. Male nursing students have reported that their fear of being falsely accused of sexual assault when they touch their patients creates an important barrier to their learning to become nurses. Male students have also reported frustration that their teachers and classmates don't recognize their challenges or help them in overcoming any conflicts they have with caring or with touch.

I recommend that you use the information provided in this chapter to help you develop your own style of caring. When you have uneasiness about caring activities, think about what might be causing your discomfort. Is there a masculinity message involved? Is there more than one message? Can you reject, revise, or reprioritize those messages? Talk openly about your conflicts with your teachers and classmates. The purpose of talking with others is not to imply that you can't do the caring. Instead, the purpose is to help them become more aware of the negotiation process, and that you are working on developing a way to work through the conflicts and provide care to others. Seek help from male role models, such as male classmates or male nurses. Ask them how they worked through the conflicts. They may have revised or reprioritized the same messages in a way that will work for you. Intimate touch creates especially difficult conflicts for many male students. Follow our techniques so that you can reduce your discomfort with intimate touch. The techniques take some practice. In time, you will find they become a natural fit for you. The techniques will become part of your own caring style.

In short, you are a caring individual, and caring is masculine. Therefore, you are a good fit for nursing. The way you care may be slightly different than others, but as you develop your own caring style, look for ways of caring that feel comfortable for you and meet the goals of patient comfort and well-being. Over time, you will see that your caring style deepens. You will learn to adjust your caring for different kinds of patients. Adjustments will happen smoothly, without much notice from you, but the caring will be there, and the caring will be the right type of caring for your patient.

REFERENCES

Benner, P., & Wrubel, J. (1989). *The primacy of caring: Stress and coping in health and illness.* Menlo Park, CA: Addison-Wesley.

Boughn, S. (2001). Why women and men choose nursing. *Nursing and Health Care Perspectives, 22*(1), 14–19.

Cancian, F. M., & Oliker, S. J. (2000). *Caring and gender.* Thousand Oaks, CA: Pine Forge Press.

Chinn, P. L., & Kramer, M. K. (2008). *Integrated theory and knowledge development in nursing* (7th ed.). St. Louis, MO: Mosby/Elsevier.

Clifford, C. (1995). Caring: Fitting the concept to nursing practice. *Journal of Clinical Nursing, 4*(1), 37–41.

Dahlberg, K. (1994). The collision between caring theory and caring practice as a collision between feminine and masculine cognitive style. *Journal of Holistic Nursing, 12*(4), 391–401.

Edwards, S. C. (1998). An anthropological interpretation of nurses' and patient perceptions on the use of space and touch. *Journal of Advanced Nursing, 28*(4), 809–817.

Estabrooks, C. A. (1987). Touch in nursing: A historical perspective. *Journal of Nursing History, 2*(2), 33–49.

Estabrooks, C. A. (1989). Touch: A nursing strategy in the intensive care unit. *Heart & Lung, 18*(4), 392–401.

Estabrooks, C. A., & Morse, J. M. (1992). Toward a theory of touch: The touching process and acquiring a touching style. *Journal of Advanced Nursing, 17*(4), 448–456.

Evans, J. A. (2002). Cautious caregivers: Gender stereotypes and the sexualization of men nurse's touch. *Journal of Advanced Nursing, 40*(4), 441–448.

Fisher, L. M., & Joseph, D. H. (1989). A scale to measure attitudes about nonprocedural touch. *Canadian Journal of Nursing Research, 21*(2), 5–14.

Gilligan, C. (1982). *In a different voice: Psychological theory and women's development*. Cambridge, MA: Harvard University Press.

Gilloran, A. (1995). Gender differences in care delivery and supervisory relationship: The case of psychogeriatric nursing. *Journal of Advanced Nursing, 21*, 652–658.

Gleeson, M., & Higgins, A. (2009). Touch in mental health nursing: An exploratory study of nurses' views and perceptions. *Journal of Psychiatric and Mental Health Nursing, 16*(4), 382–389.

Grady, C. A., Stewardson, G. A., & Hall, J. L. (2008). Faculty notions regarding caring in male nursing students. *Journal of Nursing Education, 47*(7), 314–323.

Harding, T., North, N., & Perkins, R. (2008). Sexualizing men's touch: male nurses and the use of intimate touch in clinical practice. *Research and Theory for Nursing Practice, 22*(2), 88–102.

Hart, K. A. (2005). Study: Who are the men in nursing? *Imprint, 52*(5), 32–34.

Hollinger, L. M., & Buschmann, M. B. (1993). Factors influencing the perception of touch by elderly nursing home residents and their health caregivers. *International Journal of Nursing Studies, 30*(5), 445–461.

Ieradi, J. A., Fitzgerald, D. A., & Holland, D. T. (2010). Exploring male students' educational experiences in an associate degree nursing program. *Journal of Nursing Education, 49*(4), 214–218.

Inoue, M., Chapman, R., & Wynaden, D. (2006). Male nurses' experiences providing intimate care for women clients. *Journal of Advanced Nursing, 55*(5), 559–567.

James, N. (1992). Care=organisation + physical labour + emotional labour. *Sociology of Health & Illness, 14*(4), 488–509.

Keogh, B., & Gleeson, M. (2006). Caring for female patients: The experiences of male nurses. *British Journal of Nursing, 15*(11), 604–607.

Keogh, B. J., & O'Lynn, C. E. (2007). Gender-based barriers for male student nurses in general nursing education programs: An Irish perspective. In C. E. O'Lynn & R. E. Tranbarger (Eds.), *Men in nursing: history, challenges, and opportunities* (pp. 193–204). New York: Springer.

Kidd, P. S., & Wagner, K. D. (2001). *High acuity nursing* (3rd ed.). Upper Saddle River, NJ: Prentice-Hall.

Kozier, B., Erb, G., Berman, A., & Snyder, S. (2004). *Fundamentals of nursing* (7th ed.). Upper Saddle River, NJ: Prentice-Hall.

Kramer, B. J., & Thompson, E. H. (Eds.) (2002). *Men as caregivers: Theory, research and service implications*. New York: Springer.

Le-Hinds, N. (2010). *Male nurses: Gender-based barriers in nursing school*. Unpublished dissertation, Bernard School of Education, University of the Pacific, Stockton, CA.

Leininger, M. (1991). *Culture care diversity and universality: A theory of nursing*. New York, NY: National League for Nursing Press.

Lusk, B. (2000). Pretty and powerlessness: Nurses in advertisements, 1930–1950. *Research in Nursing & Health, 23*(3), 229–236.

McCann, K., & McKenna, H. P. (1993). An examination of touch between nurses and elderly patients in a continuing care setting in Northern Ireland. *Journal of Advanced Nursing, 18*(5), 838–846.

Milligan, F. (2001). The concept of care in male nurse work: An ontological hermeneutic study in acute hospitals. *Journal of Advanced Nursing, 35*(1), 7–16.

Morse, J. M., Bottorff, J., Neander, W., & Solberg, S. (1991). Comparative analysis of conceptualizations of theories of caring. *Image: Journal of Nursing Scholarship, 23*(2), 119–126.

Morse, J. M., Solberg, S. M., Neander, W. L., Bottorff, J. L., & Johnson, J. L. (1990). Concepts of caring and caring as a concept. *Advances in Nursing Science, 13*(1), 1–14.

Mulaik, J. S., Megenity, J. S., Cannon, R. B., Chance, K. S., Cannella, K. S., Garland, L. M., & Gilead, M. P. (1991). Patients' perceptions of nurses' use of touch. *Western Journal of Nursing Research*, 13(3), 306–323.

Nightingale, F. (2003/1859). *Notes on nursing*. New York: Barnes & Noble.

Nursing and Midwifery Council. (2008). *Chaperoning*. Retrieved from http://www.nmc-uk.org/Nurses-and-midwives/Advice-by-topic/A/Advice/Chaperoning/

O'Lynn, C. E. (2004). Gender-based barriers for male students in nursing education programs: Prevalence and perceived importance. *Journal of Nursing Education, 43*(5), 229–236.

O'Lynn, C. E. (2007). Men, caring, and touch. In C. E. O'Lynn & R. E. Tranbarger (Eds.), *Men in nursing: history, challenges, and opportunities* (pp. 121–141). New York: Springer.

O'Lynn, C. E. (2010). Negotiation of constructed gender among rural male caregivers. In C. A. Winters & H. J. Lee (Eds.), *Rural nursing: Concepts, theory, and practice* (3rd ed., pp. 193–224). New York: Springer.

O'Lynn, C., & Krautscheid, L. (2011). "How should I touch you?" A qualitative study of attitudes on intimate touch in nursing care. *American Journal of Nursing, 111*(3), 24–33.

Paley, J. (2001). An archaeology of caring knowledge. *Journal of Advanced Nursing, 36*(2), 188–198.

Paterson, B. L., Crawford, M., Saydak, M., Venkatesh, P., Tschikota, S., & Aronowitz, T. (1995). How male nursing students learn to care. *Journal of Advanced Nursing, 22*, 600–609.

Paterson, B. L., Tschikota, S., Crawford, M., Saydak, M., Venkatesh, P., & Aronowitz, T. (1996). Learning to care: Gender issues for male nursing students. *Canadian Journal of Nursing Research, 28*(1), 25–39.

Reversby, S. M. (1987). *Ordered to care: The dilemma of American nursing, 1850–1945.* Cambridge: Cambridge University Press.

Riley, J. B. (2004). *Communication in nursing* (5th ed.). St. Louis, MO: Mosby.

Routasalo, P. (1999). Physical touch in nursing studies: A literature review. *Journal of Advanced Nursing, 30*(4), 843–850.

Routasalo, P., & Isola, A. (1996). The right to touch and be touched. *Nursing Ethics, 3*(2), 165–176.

Smith, J. S. (2006). Exploring the challenges for nontraditional male students transitioning into a nursing program. *Journal of Nursing Education, 45*(7), 263–269.

Solari, C. (2006). Professionals and saints: How immigrant careworkers negotiate gender identities at work. *Gender and Society, 20*(3), 301–331.

Stoller, E. (2002). Theoretical perspectives on caregiving men. In B. J. Kramer & E. Thompson (Eds.), *Men as caregivers: Theory, research and service implications* (pp. 51–68). New York: Springer.

Stott, A. (2007). Exploring factors affecting attrition of male students from an undergraduate nursing course: A qualitative study. *Nurse Education Today, 27*, 325–332.

Takase, M., Kershaw, E., & Burt, L. (2002). Does public image of nurses matter? *Journal of Professional Nursing, 18*(4), 196–205.

Thomas, C. (1993). De-constructing concepts of care. *Sociology, 27*(4), 649–669.

Thompson, E. H. (2002). What's unique about men's caregiving. In B. J. Kramer & E. H. Thompson (Eds.), *Men as caregivers: Theory, research and service implications* (pp. 20–47). New York: Springer.

Tillman, K., & Machtmes, K. (2008). Masculinity. *Men in Nursing, 3*(1), 23–28.

Tong, R. (1993). *Feminine and feminist ethics*. Belmont, CA: Wadsworth Publishing Company.

University of Colorado College of Nursing. (2008). *Caring in action: Original Center for Human Caring*. Retrieved from http://www.ucdenver.edu/academics/colleges/nursing/caring/caringinaction/Pages/caringinaction.aspx

Van Dongen, E., & Elema, R. (2001). The art of touching: The culture of "body work" in nursing. *Anthropology and Medicine, 8*(2–3), 149–162.

Wall, B. M. (2009). Religion and gender in a men's hospital and school of nursing: 1866–1969. *Nursing Research, 58*(3), 158–165.

Williams, A. (2001). A study of practicing nurses' perceptions and experiences of intimacy with nurse-patient relationship. *Journal of Advanced Nursing, 35*(2), 188–196.

Wilson, G. (2005). The experience of males entering nursing: A phenomenological analysis of professionally enhancing factors and barriers. *Contemporary Nurse, 20*(2), 221–233.

SEVEN

Landing Your First Job

Now that you have finished school and earned your degree, you are focused on getting your first job as a registered nurse (RN). But there are still a few steps to take before your first nursing paycheck. At this point, you are not yet a nurse; you are a college graduate. Although I understand the excitement students have when they finally finish school, it has always bothered me just a bit at graduation ceremonies to see students place the initials "RN" on their graduation caps. In order to legally identify yourself as an RN, you must first be licensed as an RN. Your school does not grant you a license as an RN; they grant you a college degree. Only your state board of nursing can grant you an RN license, and that license is needed to get a nursing job.

In this chapter, I will guide you through the steps you must take between graduation and your first day on the job as a nurse. Foremost, you must get your RN license. A license requires that you meet all criteria, complete all the necessary paperwork, and pass the licensure exam. At the same time, you must prepare yourself for the job search. You must secure people who will give you a reference, create your resume, complete job applications, and, of course, shine in your job interview. This time in your career can be stressful, yet exciting. With some planning, you can avoid the storms that will blow you off course, and instead, sail to your first job quickly.

THE NCLEX-RN EXAM

To get your RN license, you must first pass the National Council Licensing Examination for Registered Nurses (NCLEX-RN®). You may have thought you were done with exams once you were done with school, but this is not the case. All nursing school graduates must pass this national standardized exam conducted by the National Council of State Boards of Nursing (NCSBN) in order to get a license anywhere in the United States or her territories.

In 1994, the NCSBN adopted the computerized adaptive testing format (NCSBN, 2012a). This format allows the computer to adjust the difficulty of the exam to match the test taker's ability. This format examines your ability while you are taking the test. Based on your answers, the computer will give you questions so that you will have a 50–50 chance of getting the next question right. In other words, if you are answering questions well, the exam questions get harder. The reverse is true if you are answering questions poorly. The NCSBN believes that this format provides a more accurate evaluation of your knowledge. It also creates a shorter exam. Today, the exam has between 75 and 265 questions selected from a very large pool of questions. The computer stops the exam once it has calculated that your test performance equates to at least a 95% chance that you have exceeded or failed the passing grade. This may happen after only 75 questions, or some students may have to answer all 265 questions if their performance is very close to the passing standard (NCSBN, 2012b). Compare this to my own NCLEX-RN exam back in 1986. Back then, I had to pass five separate exams. The whole process lasted about 10 or 12 hours spread out over two days.

Most students who do well in school will do well on the NCLEX-RN exam. In 2011, 87.9% of students educated in the United States passed the exam on the first try, up slightly from 87.4% in 2010 and from 85.5% in 2007 (NCSBN, 2012c). This is good news for most students. I believe the higher rates are due to the better quality of nursing schools, increased use of standardized exams by schools (see Chapter 5), and better NCLEX-RN preparation materials and review courses available to students.

Unfortunately, for those U.S.-educated students who fail on the first try, less than 60% eventually pass the exam. Some researchers have looked at why students fail. Although each student's story is unique, researchers have identified some patterns. Students that failed the exam on the first try waited longer to take the exam, could not manage their stress and anxiety before and during the exam, and felt that they did not prepare well for the types of questions that would be asked on the exam. For example, some NCLEX-RN questions ask you to rank a list of nursing actions in order of importance for a given situation. Some NCLEX-RN questions ask you to choose multiple correct answers for one question. Some students who failed the NCLEX-RN reported that they had no practice with these types of questions in school. In addition, students who failed reported higher levels of self-doubt, less support from family and friends, and tended to think other people or situations were responsible for their poor test performance compared to students who passed the exam (Eddy & Epeneter, 2002; Poorman & Webb, 2000).

Success on the NCLEX-RN exam is more likely if you follow the test-taking tips described in Chapter 5, but Assessment Technologies Institute (ATI) offered some additional suggestions (ATI, 2010). First, be realistic about scheduling your exam. The exam is given by a private testing company (currently, Pearson VUE), which offers some flexibility in schedules. ATI recommended scheduling your exam about one month after finishing school. This gives you enough time to study your school textbooks, NCLEX-RN review programs, and other materials. They also recommended not taking the exam more than five months after school. Waiting too long can erode your confidence and tax your memory. Obviously, don't schedule your exam near stressful or disruptive events, such as weddings, vacations, or a move to a new home. Once you have your test date, try to take some time off work so you can rest and focus on the exam. ATI recommended going to the office where your test will be given a few days before your exam so that you can see where the office is located, how long it takes to get there, parking, and so on. Finally, ATI recommended that you plan your time so that you finish your study goals one full week before the test date. Spend the last week resting, doing some *light* review, and most important, building your confidence.

While waiting to take your exam, you will need to follow a well-organized study plan. Use the results of the exams you took in your nursing classes, as well as results from standardized exams, to guide you in deciding how much time to devote to each nursing topic. It would be difficult to review everything you learned in detail. Instead, focus your time on reviewing those topics that challenge you the most. Focus on concepts and principles that would apply to multiple clinical situations. For example, infection control measures are important, whether the patient is an elderly woman or a young boy. Actions to ensure effective gas exchange in the lungs are similar whether the patient has pneumonia or asthma.

When developing your study plan, invest time in some deep self-reflection. Think about what internal or external barriers might get in the way of your exam preparation. In other words, it isn't just about reviewing what you have learned that will make you successful on the exam. To be successful, you must address all barriers that may prevent successful performance. At my university, all students take a preparation class. Students reflect on their barriers and even develop a care plan for themselves—nursing diagnoses and all! For example, a student might self-diagnose himself with "Anxiety related to fear of failing an exam as evidenced by a tendency to have overly high self-expectations and past history of test anxiety." This student then examines appropriate strategies to reframe his perspectives on exams and how to avoid anxiety attacks while taking exams. We encourage students to create a daily study schedule that allows them to stay on track more easily. And be sure to remember to plan for at least a small amount of relaxation time each day. Relaxation will re-energize you physically, emotionally, and mentally.

Finally, I recommend that you also check out NCLEX-RN guidebooks in your local library or nursing school. There are many with even more tips that you might find helpful. Don't forget to read the *Candidate Handbook* from the NCSBN. This booklet gives you all the instructions you need to register and prepare for the exam, instructions on taking the exam, and how to get your exam results. Knowing what to expect will go far in reducing your stress about taking the exam. This handbook is available for free on the NCSBN website (www.ncsbn.org).

GETTING THE RN LICENSE

You are not an RN until you have your license, and only a state or territorial board of nursing can give you that license. The license protects the public and the profession from ill-prepared, incompetent, or imposter nurses (NCSBN, 2011a). Interestingly, the license is a relatively new concept for nursing. Before 1900, almost anyone could call himself or herself a nurse. As formal nursing schools developed, graduates began to call themselves *educated nurses*, but the education these nurses received varied greatly (Benefiel, 2011). In 1903, North Carolina began registering nurses (hence the name *registered nurse*). Registration was given if the nurse graduated from an approved school and passed an examination. Other states soon began registering their nurses too, but then quickly moved to a model of issuing a license. With licensure, states have more control over the qualifications for nurses and can establish legal boundaries for nursing practice. However, the old term *registered nurse* stuck since the term *nurse* was still used by others who performed some nursing tasks. Nurses who could legally practice nursing to its full extent had the authority to call themselves registered nurses. By 1923, all states provided nursing licenses. At first, licensing requirements differed from state to state. States required different minimum scores on licensing exams. In 1978, the NCSBN was formed to standardize the licensure exam nationwide (Benefiel, 2011).

In order to get a license, you must apply to a board of nursing and show that you have met all the criteria for licensure. Typically, criteria include successfully completing an approved nursing program, showing that you do not have certain criminal activities on your record, and passing the NCLEX-RN exam. If all criteria are met, you will be issued a license after paying the licensing fee. This license is your initial license, with which you can practice in that state or territory. If you move to another state, you may need to get another license for that new state. You will not have to re-take the NCLEX-RN exam, but you will have to meet all the criteria for nurses in that new state. As long as you continue to meet the criteria for a nurse's license, you can keep your license in the original state and have a license in your new state at the same time. In fact, you could have a license in many states, though this could be expensive due to licensure fees. Most states issue a license for one to two years. You must continue to meet certain work and/or education requirements in order to renew your nursing license. Of course, there is a fee each time you renew your license.

As you can see, it could be expensive to maintain a nursing license in multiple states or territories, something that is required if you work as a nurse in more than one state. In 2000, several state boards of nursing agreed to recognize each other's nursing licenses. This arrangement, called the Nurse Licensure Compact, allows nurses to work in multiple states with just one nursing license (Litchfield, 2010). Currently, 24 states participate in this program (NCSBN, 2011a). Some boards of nursing, nursing unions, and other nursing groups oppose the compact and the possibility of a national nursing license (Litchfield, 2010). Some feel that multistate licensure would lower the quality of nurses since some states have lower educational requirements for nursing than do other states. Others feel that incompetent nurses that have been disciplined in one state could easily slip across a state border to another state since they would not have to reapply for a license if they had a multistate license. Finances also play a role in this licensure debate. Many boards of nursing pay their expenses with the fees they collect for licenses.

Multistate or national licensure will cause boards of nursing to lose a revenue source. Also, unions fear that multistate licensure may make it easier for employers to hire nonunion workers.

Despite the disagreements, multistate or national licensure remains an important issue. Nurses from one part of the country need to respond to natural disasters or nursing shortages in other regions quickly, without having to apply for a new license in the affected areas. Nurses who provide consultation services or nursing care at a distance through technology (tele-health) are becoming more common. These nurses require the legal authority to work with clients in many states. Technology may bring in other licensure needs in the future. Advocates are quick to point out that the federal government already uses a multistate approach. Nurses who work for the federal government or the military are not required to have more than one nursing license, no matter where they work.

WHERE ARE THE JOBS?

Recently, students ask this question more and more. It wasn't that long ago when jobs were everywhere. Once or twice a year, my university held a career fair. Employers from all over the region would come to the fair and try to convince our students to apply for jobs. Students were enticed with sign-on bonuses, student loan forgiveness programs, and reimbursement for relocation expenses if they would only take a job. Some hospitals from areas experiencing severe nursing shortages even offered students a new car. Many students were offered jobs before they finished school (provided they passed the NCLEX-RN). Back then, if a student did not have a job shortly after graduation, it was usually because he or she wanted to take some time off before committing to a job.

Today is a very different story. Due primarily to the recent economic recession, nursing jobs are much harder to come by, especially for new nurses. As people began to lose jobs due to the recession, nurses who were working only part-time or had retired early flooded the market in order to earn incomes to support their families (Buerhaus, 2009; Buerhaus & Auerbach, 2011). Add this to today's reduced number of hospitalized patients and more students graduating from nursing schools, and it's easy to understand the tough job market for new grads (Buerhaus & Auerbach, 2011; Malone, Tagliareni, Haney, Taylor, & Mancino, 2010). One of my students who graduated in 2011 told me that she had completed over 50 job applications before she got an interview. She complained that almost every employer wanted a nurse with two or more years of experience. At a recent conference, one professor from California told me that only three of his graduating students had a job at graduation.

There are nursing jobs for new graduates, despite the doom and gloom; however, these jobs take longer to find than in the past. For example, in Washington State, 17% of new graduates from a large university nursing program had job offers upon graduation in 2010 (down from 76% in 2004) (Hirsch, 2011). Still, 58.7% of graduates found jobs within three months of graduation, and another 20.5% found jobs within six months. Almost 70% of the new nurses reported that they were satisfied with their jobs. Of those that weren't satisfied, most were unhappy with their salaries or benefits. Nationally, the forecast may be better than in Washington. The American Association of Colleges of Nursing (AACN) reported that 88% of graduates from baccalaureate programs had jobs within six months of graduation (AACN, 2011). Clearly, employment opportunities vary from location to location. Malone et al. (2010) suggested that you consider relocating to where jobs are more plentiful, if possible, after graduation.

In 2010, the Oregon Center for Nursing (OCN) surveyed health employers across the state. Only 39% of the hospitals and hospital systems were recruiting new graduate nurses (OCN, 2011). Hospitals reported only a 3.3% vacancy rate and a 7.0% turnover rate in RNs, down significantly from 2004. The main reason for the low vacancy rates were nurses working more hours or delaying retirement. However, the OCN reported that the need for nurses in hospitals continues to grow. In fact, 79% of hospitals had open positions, but many of these hospitals were seeking only experienced nurses. If hospitals were hiring new graduates, most preferred graduates with a bachelor's degree. In 2010, 71% of hospitals hoped to increase the number of nurses with bachelor's degrees. Consistent with national trends and recommendations from the Institute of Medicine, you should strongly consider earning your bachelor's degree in nursing in order to secure and maintain a job as an RN.

The OCN also looked at employment opportunities in long-term care, home health/hospice, and public health (OCN, 2011). All of the public health and long-term care employers were recruiting new graduates for vacant positions. The 2010 vacancy rate for nurses was 5.1% in public health and 4.4% in long-term care, higher than the hospital rate. Public health departments have a preference for nurses with bachelor's degrees. Long-term care employers reported a turnover rate of 21.6% in 2010, down from 26.3% in 2004 (OCN, 2011). Some nurses leave long-term care to take hospital jobs that offer higher wages, but the OCN reported that many nurses leave because they were not well prepared by their nursing schools to work in long term care. Specifically, many students do not learn the complexities of caring for the elderly and the management and administrative skills necessary for working in long term care (Reinhard, Barber, Mezey, Mitty, & Peed, 2002; Williams, Nowak, & Scobee, 2006), even though the Institute of Medicine reported that caring for the elderly in nonhospital settings is a priority need in the United States (Auerbach, Buerhaus, & Staiger, 2011). Long-term care employers are recruiting nurses with associate and diploma degrees, though more employers are preferring nurses with bachelor's degrees (OCN, 2011). In Oregon, none of the home health/hospice providers were hiring new graduate nurses. The 2010 vacancy rate in these settings was 5.9% with a turnover rate of 24.6% in 2010, the highest of the four employer types. The OCN believes that lack of support for nurses and the lack of preparation these nurses had in school for home health and hospice nursing are the primary reasons for high nurse turnover rates in these types of settings.

This information from Oregon and Washington may be different from that in your area. However, it is possible that hospital jobs may be more difficult to find than they were in the past in many locations. For example, vacancy rates for hospitals in Vermont were 5% in 2008 compared to 8% in long-term care settings (University of Vermont, 2009). Similarly, hospital vacancy rates averaged lower than those for long-term care settings in Tennessee in 2008 (Tennessee Center for Nursing, 2010). It would be wise to consider looking for jobs outside the hospital setting. Taking jobs in long-term care or public health may pose some challenges for you, particularly if your school did not prepare you well for the level of independence and management that these types of nursing careers require. However, jobs in these areas are stimulating and satisfying. In fact, the OCN (2010) reported that nurses who worked in hospitals were less satisfied with their jobs than nurses who worked in nonhospital settings. Nonhospital nurses were more satisfied with the quality of care they provided, their relationships with patients and coworkers, and their level of independence. They were less satisfied with their income than hospital nurses, but were equally satisfied with their benefits.

The economic recovery is slower than anyone would like. Not everyone is finding satisfactory jobs as soon as they had anticipated. Malone et al. (2010) offered some advice for those of you waiting for that first nursing job. First, take your NCLEX-RN exam as soon as possible. If you have a current job as a nursing assistant or other provider, keep working while you look for a job as an RN. The extra experience will be valuable; however, keep in mind that some employers will not hire you as an aide if they know that you will leave as soon as you find an RN position. What works best is to seek an aide position in the same facility you want to work in as a nurse. This situation is a win-win for you and the employer since your transition from an aide position into a nursing position will be smoother, shorter, and cheaper than someone they hire from the outside. If you chose to work as an aide, check with your local state board of nursing for any rules or regulations for RNs working as nursing assistants. Malone et al. also suggested getting volunteer, residency, or internship positions. These positions may offer lower wages, or even no wages at all, but you will gain clinical experience and keep your nursing skills current while you are looking for a job. Working in one of these positions will make you more competitive against other new nurses who are working in non–health care settings. Keep your network connections. Stay in touch with former faculty and clinical instructors. They may have job leads for you. Join a professional nursing organization. This will expand your connections while offering professional development and education opportunities at the same time. Let the members of this organization know that you are looking for a job in that specialty. Get a mentor in the field of nursing that interests you. This mentor can help you stay current in the field while keeping an eye on possible job openings. And of course, if the job search is not going well, consider using this time to further your education. Look for an associate-to-bachelor's (or master's) program. Education beyond the bachelor's degree opens up more possibilities. The OCN (2011) reported that nurses who returned to school had higher employment rates at graduation than did new graduates with bachelor's degrees. Many of these continuing programs for nurses are available online, making them convenient to your busy schedule. And most important, keep your resume and job interview skills current and professional.

LANDING THE JOB

References and the Resume

You must do two things before you start filling out job applications: find people who will give you a reference and develop a resume. First, find people you trust who will give you a meaningful reference when employers call. Some students pick the people they feel will give them the most positive references. This can be a mistake if the person cannot speak to your ability to work as a nurse. For example, I recently read an application in which the student selected a pastor as a reference. Although the pastor gave a glowing account of the student's character, the pastor could not speak to the student's clinical or professional abilities. This type of reference must be balanced by clinical references. Be sure to select faculty, advisors, nurses, and other clinicians who have observed your nursing skills and competencies. Don't forget to get permission from your references *before* you share their names with potential employers. I have been blind-sided by phone calls from employers asking about one of my former students. In these situations, I let the employer know that I had not been asked to serve as a reference, and therefore, could not provide comment on the student's ability. Also, when your reference agrees to write a reference for you, help this person by sharing your strengths with that person. It is helpful to send this person a copy of your resume to give them a better picture of your qualifications.

Your resume is possibly one of the most important written works you will complete. It must be brief, no more than two pages, yet meaningful. Your resume must help you stand out from the rest of the applicants without coming off as too showy or unprofessional. There are possibly hundreds of resume templates available on-line or at your school's career center. Recently, I looked through some resume templates I found on the Internet. Most looked very professional, and some even catered to people looking for health careers. I felt some templates were over-the-top, with borders that were too fancy or wild in color. Your resume should reflect your individual style and be visually pleasing, but it should still present a moderately conservative and professional appearance. Don't be garish in your attempt to stand out from other applicants.

Once you have selected the style of the resume, you need to carefully consider the wording. Everything on your resume should be accurate. Your resume is not a place to exaggerate your accomplishments. Instead, your resume should offer a true reflection of the strengths you might bring to the employer. Everything on your resume should be spelled correctly with no grammatical errors. Your resume should reflect your best writing ability. It's a good idea to have one of your teachers, career counselors, or peers to proofread your final draft.

Your resume should detail professional competencies and not hands-on clinical skills. Frequently, I see resumes that list the locations of where a student completed clinical rotations followed by the hands-on skills that were demonstrated at these sites (e.g., hanging IVs, inserting catheters, etc.). This approach is not effective because nursing is not a collection of tasks. Plus, clinical skills you mastered in a pediatric rotation, such as vision screens, may have little relevance to an employer who has a vacancy on a geropsych unit. Instead, highlight one or two professional competencies that you developed in each of these settings. These competencies include critical thinking, conflict resolution, interdisciplinary team communication and team building, application of evidence-based practice, participation in quality improvement initiatives, client teaching, delegation, care planning for multiple complex clients, client advocacy, professionalism, ethical decision-making, prioritization, leadership, and professional development, among others. All of these competencies are applicable to *any* RN position. So, in the pediatric example above, perhaps you worked with many low-income families and assisted the social worker and others to refer families to community resources. You could include in your resume something like, "I collaborated with social service providers to improve access to health resources for vulnerable low-income families." This type of a statement *would* have direct relevancy to clients on a geropsych unit. Remember to keep these descriptions short, no more than one or two sentences. You can discuss these competencies in more detail during the job interview, as well as describe the hands-on skills you developed if asked by the interviewer. Be prepared to explain how specific activities apply to the job you are seeking.

Finally, make sure that your resume is easily adaptable. In today's job market, you are likely to apply to several, and possibly many, different employers. Each of these employers is different. Just as you would not use the same care plan for every patient, you should *not* use the same resume for each employer. Your resume should be individualized to each employer as necessary. For example, resumes typically have a beginning statement of purpose or objective. This statement describes why you are applying for a job with that employer. This statement should be compatible with the mission statement and/or values of the employer. Research these on the employer's website. Let's say you are applying to a public health clinic that primarily serves immigrant communities. The clinic's mission statement might read, "To provide high quality health services to vulnerable members of our community in a manner that respects the inherent value and dignity of each person." You might develop a resume statement like, "Objective: To obtain an entry-level RN position that will afford me the opportunity to serve and advocate for clients and families who are most in need." You would then want to make sure that the professional competencies you highlight in your resume are those that would be most important for this kind of objective. If you speak a foreign language or have other relevant skills, you should make sure that these are stated on your resume. (*Note*: Obviously, your statement of objective should also be compatible with your own values. If you simply state something that agrees with the employer's mission statement but is *not* true for yourself, your statement will be dishonest and will be obvious to the employer during the job interview.) Electronic copies of your resume make it easy to individualize your resume. When making revised copies of your resume to give to different employers, make sure that you proofread the resume before submitting it. You don't want to have a resume that has inappropriate portions that were copied and pasted from a different resume in error.

The Application

Many employers require that you submit applications electronically. Employers find it easier to sort through electronic applications and reject those that do not meet the requirements for the job. For the applicant, electronic applications are more convenient, in that you can access them from home. Electronic applications have the ability for you to attach additional documents, such as a resume, cover letter, or certificates. But electronic applications have some drawbacks. You must make sure that you fill out all the electronic fields before you hit the "Submit" button. Forgetting to complete a field may result in your file being rejected, even though you may be well-qualified for the position. Some employers use a third party to develop and administer the electronic applications. If you have questions about the application, you may be directed to a person from the application company and not the employer. This person may not be helpful, since he or she may not be familiar with information specific to the employer. Also, some electronic applications do not allow alternative information in certain sections. This creates a "square peg in a round hole" situation. For example, some students at my university come in with prior degrees. They bypass the bachelor's degree and earn a master's degree in nursing. Although they are more educated than our baccalaureate graduates, they cannot check the "BSN" box on the electronic application. Some of the applications don't allow for a different option for the nursing degree, resulting in the rejection of their files from employers requiring a BSN degree. This has created much anxiety for students and forced us to call employers and explain our school's program. Some employers have been able to create a free-text space to allow students to explain their situations, but often software programs will not sort files by words in the free text fields. We are still trying to work through this mess.

If you are filling out paper applications, make sure that your application is filled out neatly. Never use white out on the application or cross out mistakes. This will make the application look sloppy. Instead, it's a good idea to make several photocopies of the application form before you fill it out. This will give you additional blank copies if you make a mistake while filling out the application. If you are filling out the application at the employment site, make sure you bring all necessary information with you, such as phone numbers and addresses of former employers, references, and schools. Before delivering or mailing the application, make sure you have all required attachments, such as a cover letter, resume, or other documents. Sometimes, pages get separated by the employer. Make sure that all pages include your name, whether in the title of the document or as a header, just in case one of the pages goes missing. If you hand-deliver the application, make sure it is in a cover folder or envelope with your name, date, and position you are applying for printed on the outside. If you mail the application, make sure it has the correct postage and is addressed to the right person or department.

The Interview

Up to this point, the resume and the application have introduced you to a potential employer. It's during the interview, though, where you close the deal. Here, you explain who you are and your qualifications in greater detail. Employers will have many questions for you during the interview to see if you really are the right person for the job. On the other hand, you have the opportunity to interview the employer as well during the interview. You can decide whether or not the employer is the right match for your career goals.

There are many guides and resources to help you understand what to expect at the interview. Many schools have a career center where staff works with you on developing your interview skills, including videotaping a mock interview so that you can watch yourself and spot any destructive nonverbal behaviors. Today, the typical employer uses a behavioral interview. This type of interview requires you to describe how you responded (or behaved) to certain situations in your past. For example, you might be asked how you resolved a conflict with a coworker or how you demonstrated professionalism in your clinical experiences. In order to be successful with this type of an interview, LaMaster and Larsen (2010) recommended that you think of good, but true, examples of certain situations and prepare a *brief* discussion about them. Specifically, think of situations that speak to conflict, teamwork, flexibility, communication, and taking initiative or leadership on something. They suggested following the SHARE model for discussing a situation. "S" stands for situation; describe it *briefly*. "H" stands for hindrances; describe the challenges. "A" stands for the action you took. "R" stands for the results of your actions; and "E" stands for the evaluation or summary of what you learned from this experience. As you chose some experiences to highlight, make sure you review the employer's mission statement and values. Ideally, your examples will support or be congruent with the mission and values.

Heather Lary of Providence Health System in Portland, Oregon, told me recently that most employers can teach new nurses hands-on skills such as dressing changes or programming an IV pump if necessary. It's not easy, however, to teach good time management, critical thinking, and effective teamwork. New nurses should be prepared to describe how they have already developed these professional competencies. Ms. Lary also shared that employers can spot false stories and bragging right away. Don't stretch the truth at all, period. Demonstrate compassion during the interview. Explain how you showed a caring attitude toward others, not just to patients, but to other students, visitors, or anyone else. Compassion toward classmates might suggest to an employer that you will be compassionate and supportive of future coworkers. Also, plan to describe a situation where you did something wrong, what you did to fix the problem, and what lesson you learned from your mistake. Most of all, explain what client-centered care means to you. Convince the interviewer that you truly believe that the client comes first. Table 7.1 summarizes tips you should keep in mind when you are invited to interview with an employer.

TABLE 7.1   Interview Tips

- Confirm the date, time, and location of the interview. If possible, practice driving or taking the bus to the location beforehand at the same time of day so you can see how long it takes to get there
- Practice discussing your stories with a friend or family member
- Wear business attire to the interview
- Arrive 15 minutes early to the interview
- Bring extra copies of your resume and a list of at least three references
- Greet your interviewer with a smile and confident handshake
- Speak clearly during your interview
- Listen attentively to the interviewer
- Maintain good eye contact
- Don't share any negative attitudes you have about your school, teachers, former employers, or coworkers
- Let the interviewer know that you are eager to learn and eager to contribute to the team
- Be prepared to ask your interviewer two to three questions about the employer
- Be prepared to discuss why you are the best person for the job and what sets you apart from other applicants
- Avoid asking about salary or benefits during the first interview—save that for the follow-up meeting
- Relax, smile, and be yourself

Source: Adaptation from Gaffney & Roe, 2011; LaMaster & Larsen; Sohnen-Moe, 2008.

Remember to interview the employer as well, but don't ask too many questions. (You don't want to do a complete role reversal.) However, a *few* meaningful questions suggest that you are very interested in the job. Some important questions to ask include: "Do you have a residency program for recent nurse graduates?" "What are the RN turnover and vacancy rates?" "How are nurses held accountable for high-quality practice?" "What supports are given to encourage professional development and continuing education for RNs?" "Do nurses have input when policies are developed?" The American Association of Colleges of Nursing (AACN) provides a free brochure of possible interview questions new nurses should ask potential employers (*What Every Nursing Student Should Know When Seeking Employment*, n.d.). It is available on their website at http://www.aacn.nche.edu/publications/hallmarks.pdf.

At the end of the interview, thank the interviewer. Let the interviewer know that you are eager to join the team. Ask for the interviewer's business card and remind him or her how to contact you. Ask when you should expect to hear from them. The next day, send the interviewer a thank you note. Do *not* email the note; the interviewer is probably overburdened with many emails already. A hand-written note that has been mailed shows that you are taking the extra time and care to send your thanks. If you have not heard by the expected date, wait a couple of more business days before calling. When you call, you may be told that they need more time to make their decision. Respect this. Do *not* call repeatedly to check on their progress. This will not show that you are eager for the job; instead, you will give the impression that you are pushy or impatient. Ms. Lary told me that this seems to be a problem she sees more with male applicants. She reported that many men come across as too aggressive, so let the employer make their decision on *their* schedule. If you are offered a different job somewhere else, feel free to contact the first employer. They will give you an indication as to whether you should accept the new job offer, or hold tight for an offer they may have for you.

A CAUTION ABOUT SOCIAL MEDIA

The number of social media sites and their popularity have exploded in recent years. I think it's fair to say that social media has changed our lives, even for those who don't use it regularly. Social media has challenged conventional communication and social etiquette. Social media has blurred the lines of privacy and created new avenues for nurses to get into trouble. The NCSBN has noted an increase in privacy violations from nurses involving the use of social media sites—so much so that it published a policy statement re-educating nurses and students on their legal and ethical responsibilities (NCSBN, 2011b). Today, I see a troubling destruction of the boundaries between professional and social communication, which may creep into the job search. This is particularly true for younger generations of nurses and students. Let me give you a few examples.

My partner is a supervisor at a local packaging operation. He is responsible for hiring new employees. When a position comes open, he receives a number of applications. Part of his screening process includes running an Internet search on each applicant. He finds online profiles, blogs, and other media tied to the applicant and reads them. He recently rejected the application of someone whose blog was filled with stories about parties, drinking, and late-night antics. A few nurse managers have told me that they do the same. Another example I found incredible came from a student. She told me that she had "friended" a nursing organization, a local hospital, and several nurses she met in clinical as a way to keep up a network of possible job contacts. She also included her blog contact in her professional resume. This seemed like a good idea until I asked her who her other "friends" were and what kinds of postings were accessible among friends on this site and on her blog. The look on her face made me think that she would now remove her professional friends from the site and revise her resume. A third example comes from another student. A student was angry at one of her teachers. She trashed her teacher online with multiple negative and personal comments. One of her friends posted it on her own site, sharing the comments to a whole new group of friends. One of the new friends pasted and clipped the comments and sent them via email to the teacher. The teacher filed an integrity complaint against the student, which became a part of the student's academic file.

Remember, *nothing* online is truly private. The advice, "Don't put anything online that you wouldn't be willing to publish in the newspaper" is wise. You must keep separate your professional and your social lives; otherwise, you might put yourself in a very vulnerable position in a competitive job search. Before completing applications and giving interviews, clean up your accessible online profiles. Run an Internet search on yourself and see what comes up. If possible, create an alias to communicate socially and use your legal name as your professional online presence. Don't allow yourself to be blindsided by questions from potential employers about anything embarrassing they might find online.

SUMMARY

The time immediately following graduation is filled with intense emotions. Nearly every student worries that he or she will not pass the NCLEX-RN. The good news is that a large majority of students pass the exam on the first try. To increase your chance of success, you will need to reduce your stress about the exam. The best way to reduce that stress is to be as prepared as you can be. Preparation takes some work. This chapter reviewed common tips to prepare for the exam, but these tips will be useless if you do not use them. Likewise, the job search can be very stressful as well. I must admit, I did not experience much stress finding my first nursing job. Jobs were plentiful then. Perhaps someday soon, nursing jobs will again be plentiful. For now, finding the appropriate job takes some work and some planning. Be smart on how you approach the job search. Maintain complete professionalism and be mindful on how to keep yourself as qualified and knowledgeable as possible.

Lastly, please remember that your first nursing job is just that: your *first* job. Few seasoned nurses are still working in the same job they had when they graduated from school. I find too many of my students think of their first job as the endpoint of their career journeys, when in fact, their first job is only a starting point. Others fear that their careers will be derailed if they take the wrong first nursing job. This kind of thinking is destructive. A nursing job in *any* setting affords you opportunities to learn and develop your professional competencies further. The only wrong first job is one that will not allow you to grow. These types of jobs are out there, but they are few and far between. Usually, it is you, the new employee, who hampers your own professional development and career advancement. In Chapter 9, I will discuss how to prevent self-sabotage of your career. In the meantime, embrace your first job and take advantage of every learning opportunity it provides you!

REFERENCES

American Association of Colleges of Nursing (2011). *New AACN data on nursing enrollments and employment of BSN graduates*. Retrieved from http://www.aacn.nche.edu/news/articles/2011/11enrolldata

Assessment Technologies Institute (2010). *Ready-set-RN: Preparing for the NCLEX-RN*. Stillwell, KS: Author.

Auerbach, D. I., Buerhaus, P. I., & Staiger, D. O. (2011). Registered nurse supply grows faster than projected amid surge in new entrants ages 23–26. *Health Affairs, 30*(12), 2286–2292.

Benefiel, D. (2011). The story of the nurse licensure. *Nurse Educator, 36*(1), 16–20.

Buerhaus, P. I. (2009). The shape of the recovery: Economic implications for the nursing workforce. *Nursing Economics, 27*(5), 336–340.

Buerhaus, P. I., & Auerbach, D. I. (2011). The recession's effect on hospital registered nurse employment growth. *Nursing Economics, 29*(4), 163–167.

Eddy, L. L., & Epeneter, B. J. (2002). The NCLEX-RN Experience: Qualitative interviews with graduates of a baccalaureate nursing program. *Journal of Nursing Education, 41*(6), 273–278.

Hirsch, A. M. (2011). Report of survey results for newly licensed registered nurses in Washington State. *Journal of Nursing Education, 50*(10), 575–578.

LaMaster, M. A., & Larsen, R. A. (2010). Prepare for a behavioral interview, then ace it! In *Lippincott's 2010 Nursing Career Directory* (pp. 8, 10). Ambler, PA: Lippincott.

Litchfield, S. M. (2010). Update on the nurse licensure compact. *AAOHN Journal, 58*(7), 277–279.

Malone, B., Tagliareni, E., Haney, K., Taylor, C., & Mancino, D. (2010). Your first position in nursing: Realities of the current job market. *Imprint, 57*(3), 32–34.

National Council of State Boards of Nursing (2011a). *What you need to know about nursing licensure and boards of nursing*. Chicago, IL: Author.

National Council of State Boards of Nursing (2011b). *White paper: A nurse's guide to the use of social media*. Chicago, IL: Author.

National Council of State Boards of Nursing (2012a). *2012 NCLEX examination candidate booklet*. Retrieved from http://www.ncsbn.org/1213.htm

National Council of State Boards of Nursing (2012b). *NCLEX psychometric frequently asked questions*. Retrieved from https://www.ncsbn.org/2323.htm#Last_easy_fail

National Council of State Boards of Nursing. (2012c). *NCLEX pass rates*. Retrieved from https://www.ncsbn.org/1237.htm

Oregon Center for Nursing (2010). *Career satisfaction among Oregon's registered nurses: A report from the Oregon Center of Nursing*. Portland, OR: Author.

Oregon Center for Nursing (2011). *Nurses wanted: The changing demand for registered nurses in Oregon*. Portland, OR: Author.

Poorman, S. G., & Webb, C. A. (2000). Preparing to retake the NCLEX-RN: The experiences of graduates who fail. *Nurse Educator, 25*(4), 175–180.

Reinhard, S. C., Barber, P. M., Mezey, M., Mitty, E. L., & Peed, J. A. (2002). *Initiatives to promote the nursing workforce in geriatrics*. Washington, DC: John A. Hartford Foundation.

Tennessee Center for Nursing (2010). *2010 Tennessee nursing status report*. Retrieved from http://www.centerfornursing.org/research/InfoBriefs/2010TNnursingStatus Report.pdf

University of Vermont (2009). *2009 reports: Vermont Health Workforce Assessment Survey*. Retrieved from http://www.choosenursingvermont.org/research/2009.php

What every nursing student should know when seeking employment. (n.d.). Washington, DC: American Association of Colleges of Nursing.

Williams, K. N., Nowak, J., & Scobee, R. L. (2006). Fostering student interest in geriatric nursing: Impact of senior long-term care experiences. *Nursing Education Perspectives, 27*(4), 190–193.

EIGHT

Communication: Do I Really Have to Talk About Baby Showers?

Renee G. Heath

The question posed in the title of this chapter might strike a familiar chord with many male nurses. Yet this question points to something much broader, which becomes the focus of this chapter: Why should male nurses pay attention to communication in the workplace? Communication is often overlooked in the workplace. When budgets are tight, training for such things is frequently the first thing to go out the window. Yet communication matters. When nursing skills are equal, communication can be the difference between getting promoted and not getting promoted. Sometimes poor communication skills can lead to termination. Communication creates the relationships and environments in which we live and work (think good or bad marriages or personal relationships). And, communication has very little to do with our intentions. For example, I recently sent a packet of lecture notes to be copied by our campus print shop. In the "date needed" space, I wrote ASAP, knowing that I was really late in getting my materials to the shop. My intention was that the print shop personnel would get to it as soon as they could—or literally, as soon as was possible. However, staff in the print shop interpreted my "ASAP" as "rush." They were quite peeved that I had the audacity to write ASAP when it was I who was late. Both interpretations of ASAP were correct. But the damage had been done. The new director of the campus print shop did not have a good first impression of me. I won't ever have the opportunity to take that back, despite my intentions to be more sensitive in the future. Thus, getting communication right can help us avoid situations like mine and make work a more rewarding experience.

So what about the added complexity of getting communication right between the sexes? Countless books and articles have been published on the topics of gender and communication. You probably want me to tell you that, yes, you do communicate differently from women. After all, aren't men from Mars and women from Venus (Gray, 2004)? The truth is a bit more complicated than that. Research is often mixed and inconclusive when it comes to gendered communication. I taught a gender communication course for years. Probably the most disappointing conclusion for students was that for as many studies that suggest significant gender differences, there are as many studies that suggest very little differences in gendered communication. For example, while women are often thought to talk more than men, some studies have found men actually talk *more*, for example, in the workplace (Pullen & Barrett, 2008).

"But wait," you say, "I know men communicate differently from women, I've experienced it!" Indeed you have, but those differences are more pronounced in certain *contexts,* or situations. If you examine studies on gender/ sex and communication, the studies almost always occur in a certain context. Assumptions that the findings would work in different contexts don't hold up. And it is those contexts that matter more when it comes to becoming communication competent. Bakke (2010) explained what it means to be a competent communicator:

> Communication competence is a matter of degree. It is not an absolute because there are multiple levels of appropriate and effective interpersonal situations. Interactants perceive a competent communicator to be relaxed, empathetic, supportive, and able to change their communication practice depending on the interpersonal encounter. (Wiemann, 1977, cited in Bakke, 2010, p. 349)

Therefore, to be competent at communication we need to be highly sensitive to how we are heard, the contexts in which we communicate, and the history that exists between the communicators. So to answer the pressing question asked in the title of this chapter, regarding whether you have to talk about that baby shower, I'll first discuss communication environments. These environments include the communities in which you work as nurses (communities of practice), the culture of your workplace, the styles you prefer, and how those styles need to change depending on the communication context. Next I'll discuss the provoking topic of power. Finally, the chapter will finish with some hints for detecting workplace bullying. Talking about baby showers is a matter of choice. But understanding these concepts will help you understand the choice and increase your communication skills so that you can better control the outcome of your choice.

COMMUNICATION ENVIRONMENT: COMMUNITIES OF PRACTICE

As a nurse, you belong to several communities of practice (Wenger, 1998). For example, nursing has a standard of practice to which all nurses must follow, such as laws about patient confidentiality. The customs and legal aspects of nursing practice create one type of community of practice. This community may differ from the communities of practice of other health care providers. For example, a student of mine studied the communication of nurses and doctors in an intensive care unit at a local hospital. She noted the differences in the way nurses and physicians communicated when discussing patients. From interviews with physicians, she learned that they were frequently annoyed to have long drawn out descriptions of the patients' conditions. Nurses, she noted, described the patients based on their histories and the relationships they had developed with them. Nurses sometimes used stories to describe the medical situation. At the same time, physicians complained they wanted a to-the-point description of the medical problem. This communication dilemma between physicians and nurses is best described as being influenced by their different communities of practice. It makes complete sense that nurses would describe the patient more completely, as it is their job to learn everything about their patients. Physicians, on the other hand, often need only information that they can use to diagnose the problem efficiently. Poor communication is so important that the Institute of Medicine identified it as the cause of many medical errors (Institute of Medicine, 1999). Standard protocols, such as SBAR (situation-background-assessment-recommendations) are now commonplace as a way to improve communication between physicians and nurses (Beckett & Kipnis, 2009).

Communities of practice can be even more complex when you account for different specialties in the nursing profession, such as surgical, labor and delivery, and emergency nursing. Specialty nurses have also developed particular practices, standards, and identities that distinguish them from other types of nurses. Still other communities of practice, such as those based on your gender or sex, are ingrained into us at an early age and stay with us throughout our lives. For example, baby showers are a traditional celebration that women practiced even prior to becoming nurses. It is a community of practice that has long roots. We bring multiple communities of practice with us into the workplace. What is important to understand is that if we are to get communication right and increase our communication competence, we need to be sensitive to the many communities of practice to which we belong, and the communities of practice of our coworkers.

Many scholars and writers discuss the hierarchical nature of communication between physicians and nurses. Later, I will discuss some of the complex reasons for adopting hierarchical styles of communication, but now it is important just to recognize that this type of communication is downward: physician to nurse, head nurse to staff nurse, nurse to aide. Since female nurses outnumber male nurses, communities of practice involving gender also become important in nursing.

Sensitivity to your own community of practice will help you develop sensitivities to your communication environment. Use the questions below to understand your nursing communities of practice and increase your communication competence.

1. What practices are common throughout nursing?
2. What do all nurses know? (Things that wouldn't change from place to place.)
3. What practices are typical in my specialty of nursing? How do we talk to each other?
4. How do we expect to be talked to?
5. How might this be different from other communities of practice?

COMMUNICATION ENVIRONMENT: CULTURE

Culture helps explain behavioral patterns particular to place. A hospital can have a particular culture, as can different units or floors in the same hospital. Sometimes the subculture of a unit may be stronger than the hospital culture. Usually, management will try and control culture as a way to control behavior. For example, management may encourage exercising on hospital time as a way to create a culture of healthy staff. Culture is a catch-all concept that helps us understand how we may have different languages (i.e., word choice), rituals (i.e., baby showers), and values (i.e., how to care for a patient or how to schedule staff) (Packanowski & Trujillo, 1983). Nurses who share a community of practice with each other also share a *culture* with others who may not share their community of practice. Physicians, administrators, patients, and nurses all contribute to a particular culture of a pediatric unit.

Sometimes systemic communication problems can be related to a culture within the workplace. For example, my family's general practitioner is a nice guy, but we continuously find ourselves battling his scheduling and billing staff. Even though we have been with him several years, we continue to feel frustrated with the way we are treated. I believe it is a problem of culture. The office personnel treat the patients in an aloof manner because the office structures, practices, and patterns of communication facilitate aloofness. Even though it is a small office, they sit behind large Plexiglas windows. They do not open the windows or grant you eye contact when you arrive. You must wait patiently for the staff to acknowledge your presence before they finally open the glass barrier and validate your arrival. The office structure contributes to the norms for behavior and communication. Because the staff are shielded behind the glass, they do not have to acknowledge people as they enter the office. Eye contact and a friendly hello are unnecessary until the all-important glass shield is opened, giving the message to the patient, "you are not important until I am ready to greet you." This attitude permeates all aspects of his office and his practice. Contrast this with my sister who is a physical therapist. She has built a satisfied clientele based on her reputation for treating patients so well. Clients enter a warmly decorated office and are at once greeted and offered a homemade espresso or latte. Cookies and biscotti are always out for waiting patients to help themselves. The message to the patient is that they are important, their time is valuable, and their comfort is considered. All of these "messages" are embedded in the culture of the offices, largely created by physical structures, behaviors, and rituals.

Culture and communities of practice intersect when you enter a unit that ritually celebrates babies and marriages with cakes and parties. This ritual may not be present in all settings. For example, some units may find themselves too busy to have time to plan celebrations. I remember working as a development director for a nursing home and finding it odd that staff celebrated every milestone in their colleagues' lives—graduations, babies, and marriages. It was not a ritual I was familiar with. I had previously worked in nonprofit and government organizations that employed more men than this nursing home. Typically, the only ritual was going out for happy hour drinks. However, the mostly female nursing home staff, which was also mostly baby-boomer in age, carried out the practice of celebration as a ritual. I eventually came to appreciate their desire to celebrate the human aspects of our lives in the workplace. And in a very real way, one of those graduation parties inspired me to go back to school for my doctoral degree.

Increasing your sensitivity to the culture of your workplace will naturally increase your communication competence. While gender plays a part in the historical customs of some of the things you experience as a male nurse (as discussed in Chapter 3), the workplace culture also plays an important role in whether or not negative experiences continue for male nurses. Rather than viewing communication problems narrowly through the lenses of gender and sex differences, consider the more complex ways communities of practice and culture intersect in your work environment to influence the rituals, practices, and languages that are dominant in your workplace. To examine your work culture, reflect on the questions below:

1. How does it feel to work in this unit?
2. What practices contribute to this feeling?
3. Which norms are unique to this unit? Do we buy each other coffee? Do we socialize outside of work?
4. How do people talk to each other in this unit? How is this different or the same than other places I've worked?

COMMUNICATION ENVIRONMENT: COMMUNICATION STYLES

A third major concept that contributes to our understanding of the communication environment is communication styles. Styles are often connected to leadership styles. The most common leadership styles are laissez faire, democratic, and authoritarian (Hackman & Johnson, 1993). *Laissez-faire* leaders are known to be hands-off. They are not directive-driven in their communication and are more likely to offer you a goal to obtain rather than a step-by-step plan for how to get there. *Democratic* leaders are identified by their willingness to request feedback from followers, and then incorporate that feedback into the decisions they make. Democratic leaders tend to be collaborative in their interactions with others and pay great attention to communication processes. By contrast, *autocratic* leaders are less interested in gathering feedback from their followers. They tend to be very direct communicators who often make decisions independently.

Gender differences in leadership have been examined in regards to communication styles, and not surprisingly, men have been associated with more direct styles of communication (commands, use of "I" language, lack of qualifiers) while women are often associated with more collaborative styles of communication (requests rather than commands, use of "we," tendency to qualify or hedge as in "I know you are busy but"). There are many possible theories for this but most scholars agree that women and men's traditional roles in society have socialized, or taught, us to speak in particular styles. These styles have allowed men and women success in particular situations. The key phrase here is *in particular situations*. After having read the above sections, you know by now that communities of practice and culture are important intervening concepts when it comes to communication. Even masculine (direct) and feminine (collaborative) styles of communication are more or less successful depending upon the context of the communication situation.

For example, creative contexts demand that a leader's communication style encourages others to share their ideas. So if you are on a problem-solving team in your hospital that is trying to decrease infection rates, you will want those in the lead to encourage feedback, have excellent listening skills, and not be too forceful with their own ideas. This will allow for creative solutions. If you are comforting a patient or family who has just learned they have a terminal disease, your style of communication should be cautious, sensitive, and less direct. These styles of communication are frequently stereotyped as feminine, but clearly men need to be able to communicate these ways in these situations too. However, if you are in the midst of a surgical procedure, you want the communication to be direct and specific, a style that is frequently stereotyped as masculine. High stress, intense decision-making moments are not the time to encourage collaboration, or to be overly sensitive to word choice. Direct styles of communication are often needed when the task is complicated, such as a surgery, when decisions must be made quickly, or if others are not motivated or skilled to carry out the task (Hersey & Blanchard, 2008). If you are in a workplace that has a very hierarchical culture, I would suspect that the usual style of communication is autocratic, direct, and masculine. However, highly skilled persons (like nurses), or those who expect greater autonomy in their jobs do not prefer this style of communication. In fact, tolerance for direct, autocratic, and masculine styles of communication is waning as younger generations of workers expect greater autonomy and collaboration in the workplace (Martin & Tulgan, 2006).

It is important to remember that continuing to think of communication styles as masculine or feminine reinforces inaccurate stereotypes. Researchers point out that men in professions that are female-dominated (i.e., nursing and teaching) often demonstrate great skills in collaborative styles of communication. This suggests that the context of the communication may be more important than gender or sex (Stewart, Cooper, & Friedley, 1986). More importantly, different contexts demand different communication styles. Although we may find we are socialized to communicate more in one style than in another, these styles are simply patterns of communication that have become our default setting over time. In other words, we can adapt our style to different situations with practice, but it may take practice to communicate in a style that is different from our default style. If we recognize our default style and the needed style for the context of the communication, we can adjust our style accordingly.

To increase your communication competence in the workplace, consider your default style for communication. Then reflect on the questions below:

1. What is my preferred communication style at work?
2. When has this style of communication been successful?

3. When has this style of communication contributed to misunderstanding or frustration?
4. How do my coworkers perceive my style of communication?
5. What situations do I encounter that call for me to adjust my communication style?

POWER

Before you navigate the baby shower question, you need to consider another major area of communication: power. Power is both fun and controversial to talk about. Whether we recognize it or not, power undergirds most of the conflict we have both in our personal and work lives, especially conflicts between the sexes. Therefore, understanding power is an important aspect of navigating gender issues in the workplace. Communication expert Stanley Deetz (1995) argued that when we communicate we are always negotiating knowledge (what counts as truth), our own identities, our relationships with others, and grander concepts like *social orders* of society. Gender and sex issues have much to do with these important areas of communication negotiation.

The first area of negotiation—knowledge—is probably the most obvious to us. When you advocate for a certain course of action to be taken with a patient, you are negotiating what you believe is true for this patient. At the same time, you are also negotiating the second area—your identity. For example, if you are a new nurse, you are negotiating your identity as a nurse. Your communication is not only about advocating for the patient, but you are also demonstrating your knowledge as a professional. You want to be effective in establishing your *identity* as a capable nurse. How you communicate in that situation also affects the third area of negotiation—your *relationships*. If you are communicating with another nurse who responds openly to your suggestions and agrees to help you implement a course of action, then you are successfully negotiating a collaborative relationship with that nurse. If the seasoned nurse dismisses your suggestions, however, she or he is reinforcing his or her relationship with you—in this case, reinforcing his or her role as your superior. In this third area of communication we are always negotiating power. For example, if I were to come to class and say, "Today we are going to have a pop quiz!" I have communicated much more than the fact that a quiz is about to happen. I have reinforced my identity as the teacher, who has the power to implement a pop quiz. In this way, I reinforce my authority over my students.

The fourth area of communication negotiation is a bit more complicated, but even more relevant to gender/sex issues in the workplace. Every time you communicate, you are negotiating *social orders* (Deetz, 1995). In the example above, if I spring a pop quiz on my students, I am also reinforcing the hierarchy of our educational system. It would not be acceptable if the Department of Motor Vehicles surprised you one evening with a pop quiz regarding the rules of driving, but in the educational system, this imbalance of power is regularly practiced and even expected. Continuing this practice reinforces the power and hierarchy built into our educational system. Now consider yourself, a rookie male nurse, suggesting to a seasoned female nurse a new course of action for a patient. While you are indeed negotiating what you believe is true about the patient, your identity as a skilled nurse, and your relationship with this nurse, you are also negotiating social orders, and the history of social orders between men and women is complex and power laden. Sometimes this works to your benefit. Sometimes, through no fault of your own other than you were born male, you bear the brunt of your forefathers' privileged position of power (patriarchy) in our society (see Chapter 3). For example, some scholars have noted that male nurses are at times listened to more often than female nurses simply because men have held powerful roles in our society (Pullen & Barrett, 2008). For this very reason, some women may react negatively to you in response to a history of dominance from men in the home and workplace. More than likely, their response is unintentional, but it is influenced by the historical relationships, nevertheless, between men and women.

Consider another example. When I was the young development director for a skilled nursing facility, I had a male boss who repeatedly referred to me as "hon" (short for honey). I was very insulted by this term of endearment even though I am quite sure he did not mean any disrespect. At the same time, any number of the elderly patients who lived in the facility could refer to me as "hon" without incurring the same irritating reaction from me. Power is the reason that I was not bothered by the elderly patients, but I was bothered by my supervisor. Deetz's (1995) areas of communication negotiation help explain how this boils down to power. With the elderly patients, I was not threatened by the address of "hon" as it did not attack the knowledge I held as the development director, nor my identity in this role. In fact, the relationship they reinforced with me by calling me "hon" was one of closeness and friendship. The negotiation area of social orders was not involved. They were not implying that I served a subordinate role to them when they used this term. Indeed, they reinforced their roles as elders in our society, which in our culture is sadly not one of power. However, when my boss called me "hon," he reinforced a long history of unequal relationships between men and women. He would have never referred to his own boss, a woman, with this phrase. Not only was my rejection of this term a fight for my identity as a professional and as a capable peer in the field, but I rejected the entire history that ever made it okay for men to refer to women as "hon" in the workplace. As sweet as this word sounds, it is also an intimate word you use with a loved one. This made his use of the word inappropriate because I did not share an intimate friendship with him. This is why it is okay for our friends (or in my case, the elderly folks in the facility) to use terms of endearment, but it is not okay for our bosses to do so. Where power is present, certain words and phrases take on and reinforce other meanings. Like it or not, we can't escape the history of unequal relationships between the sexes, so the best way to handle these situations is to increase our sensitivity to how power works in every communication situation.

Deetz's (1995) framework helps us understand the complexity of power. When someone responds to us in an unreasonable manner, it is too easy to dismiss someone as crazy, emotional, or controlling. A smart question to ask might be, "What do I need to consider in order to believe that there might be a reason for this person's response?" (Tracy & Standerfer, 2003). We should consider the role of power in a communication situation by analyzing the various things that are being negotiated in any given communication situation. Increase your communication competence by sharpening your sensitivity to power in communication situations. Reflect on a particular communication situation you experienced with a female coworker. Use the following questions to examine how power might have influenced that situation:

1. What knowledge was negotiated? Did you agree? Did you dispute each other's facts and interpretations?
2. What identity was reinforced by you in the conversation? By her? Did you establish yourself as a capable nurse, friend, or student?
3. How would you describe the relationship that was reinforced with your conversation? Is power present and appropriate in the relationship that was reinforced or did the conversation leave you feeling more like equals, peers, or partners?
4. What role might social orders play in your communication situation? Does her response indicate she may be resisting historical orders of dominance? Were you sensitive to how she might have heard you?

BULLYING

One final important communication topic that affects all relationships is workplace bullying. Research on workplace bullying is growing in fields like psychology and communication. Workplace bullying touches most workplaces on some level. Interestingly, a tremendous amount of research on workplace bullying has been done in the field of nursing, which is reputed to have high levels of bullying behavior. Bullying is important to talk about when considering communication between men and women and should never be tolerated no matter what the sex of the bully. Lutgen-Sandvig and Tracy are communication experts on the subject of workplace bullying. They warn that bullying is a serious problem because it can lead to a variety of harmful outcomes such as psychosomatic illness, posttraumatic stress disorder, and even thoughts of suicide. Other costs associated with bullying include increased medical expenses and reduced productivity in the workplace (Lutgen-Sandvik & Tracy, 2012).

What is Bullying?

Bullying is visible in communication practices such as humiliation; spreading rumors; rude, foul, and abusive language; persistent criticism; and explosive outbursts such as yelling, screaming, and swearing (Lutgen-Sandvik & Tracy, 2012). But those behaviors alone may not be enough to constitute bullying. Other important characteristics that help you determine if you are being bullied include the intensity of the behavior (how inappropriate is the behavior?), the persistence of the behavior (how frequently does it happen?), and the power differences between those who bully and those who are bullied (are you in a position to ignore the bullying behavior or are you at the mercy of the bully?). For example, the frequency, repetition, and duration help you determine if spreading a rumor is simply inconsiderate or is actually bullying behavior. Or, if you are yelled at only rarely, it is probably not bullying; but if you have been yelled at by the same person over and over again, especially a person who holds power over you, then it is bullying (Lutgen-Sandvik & Tracy, 2012).

A Cultural Problem

Workplace culture has a lot to do with bullying. Although some people have traits and personality disorders that lead to bullying behaviors, some bullies are acting in ways they believe are acceptable in their field. That is why certain fields, like nursing, have become a hotbed for bullying behaviors. Workplaces that have hierarchal organizations so that power is concentrated by people at the top, that have intense work situations, and that have rigid procedures all create a fertile bed for bullying behaviors. People in these workplaces often dismiss bullying as "just the way it is." That said, it is difficult to make cultural changes in the workplace without having the power to do so. Therefore, it is important to learn what you can do when you encounter workplace bullying. Still, this should not discourage you from working on strategies that will make lasting changes in your workplace that will make it hard for bullying behavior to continue.

Strength in Numbers

One thing you do have the power to do is to support those who have been bullied. Experts find that communication behaviors often work to sustain bullying (Lutgen-Sandvik & Tracy, 2012). For example, silence is one communication behavior that does nothing to get rid of bullying, and indeed, may make the bullying behavior appear to be normal. Also, speaking with the boss directly about bullying is often not effective and may aggravate the bullying behavior (Lutgen-Sandvik, 2006). Researchers have found that individuals who report bullying are more likely to be blamed or suffer demotion, transferring, or firing than those who join others to report bullying as a group (Lutgen-Sandvik, 2006). Coworkers play an important part in bolstering the credibility of your claims, especially if they do not suffer from the bullying behaviors themselves, but still verify that the bullying does occur. So perhaps the first thing to consider when you encounter a bully is to find out if someone else has witnessed or experienced this behavior. A collective effort to report and change the abuse is likely to be more successful than an individual effort.

Tell a Credible Story

When reporting a bully at work, researchers recommend that you "frame stories in relatively unemotional and brief ways" so that you will be seen as professional and competent (Lutgen-Sandvik, Namie, & Namie, 2009, p. 32). Characteristics of a credible story include the following:

1. Your story should have a clear beginning, middle, and end. Be careful not to lose people with a meandering matrix of details.
2. Clearly identify the bully.
3. Focus on the bully's destructive behavior, not your response to that behavior.
4. Provide very specific detail about your bullying experience, not other smaller complaints.
5. Try and anticipate the objections that might arise and acknowledge other people's perceptions.
6. Portray a vivid description of the abuse, but avoid excessive emotion so that the person listening feels compelled to console you rather than help solve the problem.
7. Be consistent and include detailed quotes, times, places, and people.
8. Use metaphors or examples that others may find familiar.
9. Identify other people who have been bullied.
10. Provide details about the negative effects of bullying on your coworkers and the productivity of your workplace (Tracy, Alberts, & Rivera, 2007).

Craft Antibullying Policies

As you advance in your career into more administrative roles, you will be in a better position to truly help get rid of bullying. As an administrator, an important step you can take to reduce bullying is to include specific antibullying language into workplace policies (Cowan, 2009). Without these policies, administrators and human resource departments are left trying to figure out which behaviors are worthy of discipline. For example, the laws and workplace policies regarding sexual harassment have clearly defined which behaviors constitute sexual harassment. The same can be done in your organization regarding what constitutes bullying. Then when complaints are filed, individuals in positions of power have clear policies to support their decisions to discipline the bully. These policies can also work to create a culture of respect throughout the organization (Cowan, 2009).

Am I Being Bullied?

If you think you are being bullied in the workplace, take the following steps:

1. Identify the behaviors and determine if they meet one of the criteria for bullying behavior. Is the behavior frequent? Has it been going on a long time? Is it coming from a person of power? The presence of just one of these criteria might constitute bullying.
2. Consider who would be willing to support you. Are there others experiencing the same behaviors? Have others witnessed your bullying experience? Share this chapter with them and enlist them as you craft a united coalition of support.

3. Tell a credible story. Use the nine criteria above to describe your experience in a concise, yet intelligent manner. Practice the story with others who can help you better explain the confusing or fuzzy details.
4. Help your workplace craft policies against bullying by providing clear descriptions of behaviors that are unwanted and unacceptable in your field.
5. Consult and enlist other resources that can help you make your case, such as the Workplace Bullying Trauma Institute (WBI) http://www.workplace-bullying.org/. In addition, there are many books and articles about bullying that you might find helpful.

SUMMARY

Let's return to the original question that launched our thinking with this chapter: do you really have to talk about that baby shower? The answer to that question is not a clear yes or no. The answer lies in your communication competence, specifically in your ability to understand what would be the norm for other nurses in your workplace. With increased sensitivity to the work context, you can judge how your decision to discuss or not discuss that baby shower will be received by your fellow nurses. You can also use your knowledge about communication styles to engage or disengage in such a conversation. If not talking about the baby shower might offend the new mom, than you can use your collaborative nursing skills to let the new mom know you are happy for her, but that going into all the details about the baby shower is not your thing. In this case, a less directive-driven communication style would be a good choice.

However, you will also need to take into account the power dynamics of your decision to engage or not to engage in baby shower talk. If you are in charge, will your silence likely change whether future discussions about baby showers will happen in your workplace? Is reshaping the culture really what you want or would be best for teamwork? What will be gained or lost with this influence? Finally, and I say this seriously, you should never feel bullied into engaging in a practice that is unrelated to your work and makes you feel uncomfortable. In other words, if pressure to talk about baby showers is frequent, enduring, or persistent and if this pressure truly makes you feel uncomfortable, then you might be experiencing bullying behavior. In that case, enlist the support of others and use your communication competence to express how this practice is not healthy for strong relationships between the sexes in the workplace.

Final Points to Remember

1. Communities of practice affect how we communicate to one another on the job.
2. The culture of our workplace affects how we communicate on the job.
3. Communication styles need to adapt to different workplace contexts.
4. Recognize the role power plays in your conversations.
5. Bullying is not an individual problem and, therefore, requires a group response.

REFERENCES

Bakke, E. (2010). A model and measure of mobile communication competence. *Human Communication Research, 36*(3), 348–371.

Beckett, C. D., & Kipnis, G. (2009). Collaborate communication: Integrating SBAR to improve quality/patient safety outcomes. *Journal for Healthcare Quality: Promoting Excellence in Healthcare, 31*(5), 19–28.

Cowan, R. L. (2009). *Walking the tightrope: Workplace bullying and the human resource professional.* Unpublished Doctoral Dissertation, Purdue University, West Lafayette, IN.

Deetz, S. (1995) *Transforming communication transforming business: building responsive and responsible work places.* Cresskill, NJ: Hampton Press.

Gray, J. (2004). *Men are from Mars, women are from Venus: The classic guide to understanding the opposite sex.* New York: HarperCollins.

Hackman, M. & Johnson, C. (1993). The status of leadership coursework in communication. *The Michigan Association of Speech Communication Journal, 28,* 1–13.

Hersey, P., Blanchard, K. H., & Johnson, D. (2008). *Management of organizational behavior: Leading human resources* (9th ed.). Upper Saddle River, NJ: Prentice-Hall.

Institute of Medicine. (1999). *To err is human. Building a safer health system.* Washington, D.C.: The National Academies Press.

Lutgen-Sandvik, P., (2006). Take this job and …: Quitting and other forms of resistance to workplace bullying. *Communication Monographs, 73,* 406–433.

Lutgen-Sandvik, P., Namie, G., Y Namie, R. (2009). Workplace bullying: Causes, consequences, and corrections. In P. Lutgen-Sanvik & B. D. Syperh (Eds.), *Destructive organizational communication: Processes, consequences, and constructive ways of organizing* (pp. 27–52). New York: Routledge/Tayor & Francis.

Lutgen-Sandvik, P., & Tracy, S. H. (2012.) Answering five key questions about workplace bullying: How communication scholarship provides thought leadership for transforming abuse at work. *Management Communication Quarterly, 26*(1), 3–47.

Martin, C. & Tulgan, B. (2006). *Managing the generation mix: From urgency to opportunity.* New York: Human Resource Development.

Packanowsky, M. E., & O'Donnell-Trujillo, N. (1983). Communication and organizational cultures. *Communication Monographs, 50,* 126–147.

Pullen, R., & Barrett, L. (2008). Closing the communication gender gap. *Men in Nursing, 5*(3), 20–23.

Stewart, L., Cooper, P. J., & Friedley, S. A. (1986). *Communication between the sexes: Sex differences and sex-role stereotypes.* Scottsdale, AZ: Goruch Scarisbrick.

Tracy, K. & Standerfer, C. (2003). Selecting a school superintendent: Interactional sensitivities in the deliberative process. In L. R. Frey (Ed), *Group communication in context: Studies of bona fide groups* (2nd ed., pp. 109–134). Mahwah, NJ: Lawrence Erlbaum.

Tracy, S. J., Alberts, J. K., &Rivera, K. D. (2007). *How to bust the office bully: eight tactics for explaining workplace abuse to decision-makers.* Retrieved from http://humancommunicaiton.clas.asu.edu/aboutus/wellnsspublications.html

Wenger, E. (1998). *Communities of practice.* New York: Cambridge University Press.

NINE

Getting Ahead Without Stepping on Toes: Transition to Practice, Professional Development, and Leadership

Now that you have landed that job, your goal is to thrive as a new RN. For many, the first two years in nursing carries as much stress and learning as did nursing school. There are many sources for the stress, including increased responsibility placed on the shoulders of new nurses, sicker patients, unsupportive coworkers and supervisors, and increased complexities found in the workplace (National Council of State Boards of Nursing [NCSBN], 2011). In addition, employers often complain that new nurses are ill-prepared for the demands of nursing (Benner, Sutphen, Leonard, & Day, 2010). Del Bueno (2005) reported that the majority of nurse graduates lacked the ability to apply theory to practice and exercise sound clinical judgment at a beginner's level. New graduates often leave school thinking they are well-prepared for nursing practice, only to find that they have a lot of catching up in order to be safe beginning nurses. For example, more than 40% of new nurses admit to medication errors (NCSBN, 2011). Realizing that you are not as prepared for something as you thought can be incredibly stressful, and stress increases job dissatisfaction. Over 25% of new nurses leave their first job within the first year. This turnover increases health care costs and reduces the quality of patient care (Duffield, Roche, O'Brien-Pallas, & Catling-Paull, 2009; Jones 2008).

In this chapter, I will focus on ways to help you thrive as a new nurse. I will summarize Benner's novice-to-expert model (Benner, 1984; Benner, Tanner, & Chesla, 2009), a classic view on how nurses gain expertise. I will discuss effective orientation programs, especially residency programs, which ease the transition from nursing school to nursing employment. And I will discuss ways to develop your nursing competence and leadership skills. This chapter will help you find a strong footing for career satisfaction and success.

BENNER'S NOVICE-TO-EXPERT MODEL

Some 30 years ago, Patricia Benner published groundbreaking work on how nurses gain clinical expertise (Benner, 1984). Adapting a model first developed by Stuart and Hubert Dreyfus describing how chess players and airline pilots gain skill, Benner presented how clinical experience and pattern recognition help nurses become experts. Many of you are familiar with Benner's work since it has become a common topic in nursing school and professional development programs. However, Benner's work is worth reviewing. I find many students grow impatient with their progress or forget that even seasoned nurses can display beginner behaviors when they face a new challenge. You do not acquire skill overnight. It is continually developed throughout your career.

Benner's revision of the Dreyfus model has five stages. All persons go through these stages sequentially. In other words, everyone starts as a novice, but as noted above, clinical experts may have to return to an earlier stage if faced with a new situation. The first stage is the novice. The novice has no experience with the situation. He must apply book knowledge to assess and act upon the situation. He follows rigid rules and principles. He follows steps in sequence, but lacks an ability to prioritize or interpret complex findings. You may remember this stage the first few times you completed physical exams or gave medications.

The advanced beginner makes up the next stage. The advanced beginner can "demonstrate marginally acceptable performance" (Benner, 1984, p. 22). From prior clinical experiences, he begins to recognize aspects of a specific clinical situation that aid in appropriate interpretation of clinical findings. He can use guidelines and cues to help guide his clinical action, instead of having to depend upon a rigid list of rules and sequence of steps. Teachers and mentors can help his development by directing him to appropriate guidelines and discussing how he interprets and makes meaning of a situation. Depending upon the student's prior clinical experience, the new graduate enters as an advanced beginner for common clinical situations he might encounter on the job.

The next stage describes the competent nurse. This nurse begins to see things as a bigger picture. He sees how his decisions and actions contribute to long-term plans and goals. He begins to adjust and prioritize his actions to meet those goals most efficiently. In order to do this well, the competent nurse has developed perspective and a higher clinical analytic ability. Teachers and mentors can assist this nurse by guiding him through decision-making exercises and planning the care of multiple and complex patients.

Proficiency is the next stage. The proficient nurse is able to see a complete clinical picture rather quickly. He does not require a thorough collection of data because he has seen this clinical situation many times. He can determine whether or not the patient is progressing normally. He is able to pick up on very subtle clues that might indicate something in one situation, but something very different in another. For example, he is able to determine if a patient's hesitancy to get out of bed is due to pain or due to a fear of falling just by observing the patient's behaviors and facial expressions. If something isn't as expected, the proficient nurse catches the difference and acts quickly to prevent or minimize problems. Teachers and mentors can assist this nurse by using case studies in which the nurse must identify hidden clues and discuss theories and other types of knowledge that would explain why certain actions might work well or not work well. These case studies should be complex and have no definite right or wrong solution. An example might be a situation in which different treatments and actions would accomplish different desirable and undesirable outcomes, or situations that carry ethical or legal considerations.

The final stage is that of the expert. The expert nurse no longer relies on rules or guidelines. Instead, he knows when to not follow a guideline or when to break rules in order to do what's best for the patient. The expert is able to do this because he is able to recognize clinical patterns. He has seen so many cases that he knows what's going on and what to do almost immediately. His knowledge has become so engrained that he has difficulty explaining how he knew what to do. Instead, he might simply explain, "I just knew." His expertise is recognized by both patients and coworkers. What is helpful for the expert nurse is to develop a habit of reflecting back on a complex decision and identifying all the cues he used to make his clinical decisions. Detailed documentation in the patient's chart can help with this. Also, the expert should become a consultant and mentor to coworkers. In providing consultations, the expert will be pressed to explain so that others might learn from him.

The lines between Benner's stages are fuzzy. Instead of thinking these stages as distinct, you should view the stages as places on a continuum. As time goes by, you will find yourself gaining higher levels of expertise in some clinical situations, but staying at a more beginner level in other situations. With more experience, you will naturally move forward. However, Benner (1984) noted that experience isn't just gained by time on the job. Instead, experience comes with repeated and meaningful encounters with a clinical situation so that you improve your ability to see nuances. Experience results in changes in your perspective. It builds your clinical knowledge. Your forward movement will be much more meaningful if you use clinical mentors to help guide you through the experiences and necessary reflections.

Let me use my own experience as an example. I took my first RN position in 1986, two years after Benner's work was published. At that time, most of us who had attended a college or university-based nursing program had clinical experiences that were very limited in scope. Clinical time was used primarily to practice procedures we had learned. In my program, we never had opportunities to manage, lead, or delegate. We were not challenged to think critically. On top of this, few employers offered much of an orientation program. In my first job, I spent one day getting a tour of the hospital and reviewing benefits and general employee information. I spent two days working with a nurse who showed me where everything was located on the unit and explained my responsibilities. I was on my own on the third day. Two weeks later, I was charge nurse on a 24-bed neurology unit with one other nurse and one aide. I had no preceptor, no clinical mentor. Although I could ask coworkers questions, I was so busy, there was little time to discuss or reflect on what I was experiencing. In time, I gained expertise in my field, but often this expertise was gained passively, over much time, with many repeated exposures to neurology patients.

I don't think my situation was unusual for nurses of my generation. I believe many employers put new nurses to work as fast as possible in a sink-or-swim fashion. New nurses would experience clinical situations multiple times in a short period, but as Benner noted, repeating something multiple times doesn't necessarily build expertise. Benner (1984) noted that new graduates need about two or three years on the job with many clinical experiences and reflection before moving beyond the advanced beginner to the level of competence. This was probably reasonable at that time. It took me at least that amount of time before I developed competence caring for patients of varying neurological problems. Today, I think this timeframe for reaching competence can be shorter, thanks in part to improved orientation and transition to practice programs. But a faster journey to competence requires that you develop strong reflective skills and a desire to learn. It requires much work on your part. It also requires a supportive workplace and good mentorship.

TRANSITION TO PRACTICE: THE BENEFITS OF RESIDENCY

Residency programs have been used for many decades for educating doctors. Few doctors could come right out of medical school and work safely or well. In residency programs, new graduate doctors are able to practice skills, receive advanced instruction and supervision by experienced doctors, and have opportunities to discuss, reflect, and learn from difficult clinical cases. During the program, new doctors are slowly given more independence and authority as their skills and experience allow. Depending upon the specialty and location, residency programs can last from a few months to more than a year.

Residency programs for new nurses have been around at least since the 1980s, but until recently, they have been uncommon and poorly structured (Altier & Krsek, 2006). Since then, nursing practice has changed greatly. Nurses are required to assess increasingly complex patients, diagnose health and wellness conditions, think critically, make independent decisions, lead and coordinate health care teams, evaluate the effectiveness of care, engage in research and quality improvement activities, and advocate for improved health and human rights. Few new nursing graduates are able to come out of school and exercise these responsibilities much beyond a novice level. As noted earlier, this lack of preparation harms both patients and nurses. Turnover rates are high among new graduates due to the stress and dissatisfaction of a smooth transition from nursing school to nursing employment. Losing a new nurse employee is expensive too. Jones (2008) reported that the loss of one nurse can cost an employer up to $88,000 in 2007 dollars. These new realities have increased the importance for implementing residency programs for nurses.

A number of researchers have demonstrated the benefit of nurse residency programs recently. Altier and Krsek (2006) examined the effect a one-year nurse residency program had on job satisfaction and turnover rates in 316 new graduate nurses in six hospitals. They reported that job satisfaction scores were high, though lower for non-White nurses. The average turnover rate was 9.8%, much lower than published turnover rates at that time. The researchers stated that the program was a success, but that further exploration was needed on how to meet any special needs of minority nurses. A longer study was completed by Ulrich et al. (2010), who examined a nurse residency program in a hospital system over 10 years involving over 6,000 new graduate nurses. Their findings were very positive. They reported turnover rates that dropped from 24% to 7%. They noted that self-confidence among the new graduates was accelerated with the residency program. Most important, they reported that the competency level of the new graduates in the residency program after 12 months equaled the level of competency of nonresidency nurses after 17 months. In other words, residency program nurses gained competence faster than other nurses.

Studies like these have prompted the NCSBN to launch a study of its own in July 2011. This study will look at the effect of a one-year residency program for new graduate nurses in Illinois, Ohio, and North Carolina. The program will be implemented in hospitals and nonhospital settings and will be compared to other facilities not using the residency program. NCSBN will evaluate how well the program improves the quality of nursing care, increases job satisfaction, and reduces turnover. The program will use a standardized format in which new graduates work with a preceptor for six months, followed by ongoing mentorship and support for another six months. The format was developed by a team of expert clinicians, educators, and regulators and emphasizes the use of evidence-based practice to promote quality and safety. The program includes focused learning with modules and clinical activities in safety, clinical reasoning, patient-centered care, quality improvement, and informatics. Each employer has some flexibility on how to implement the modules and tailor the content appropriate to the particular clinical setting. NCSBN expects the study to be finished in 2014. They anticipate positive findings from this study that will support their vision that *all* new graduate nurses must complete a standard residency program in order to renew their nursing licenses (NCSBN, 2011).

Your employer may not be using the NCSBN model, or may not offer a residency program at all. Many employers continue to offer only a typical orientation program in which you learn policies and procedures and work with an experienced nurse for one to several weeks. Some specialty units offer a longer orientation program. Other employers offer a modified version of a residency program. Some of these programs may be effective. However, the lack of a program or even an inadequate program should not stop you from receiving the benefits of residency. The content and interactive exercises of the NCSBN Transition-to-Practice electronic modules are available for public viewing on their website (https://www.ncsbn.org/2011_TransitiontoPractice_Modules_082511.pdf). These modules, coupled with the use of clinical mentors in your clinical setting, can be valuable resources as you develop your own professional development program.

PROFESSIONAL DEVELOPMENT

The nursing code of ethics, as developed by the American Nurses Association (ANA), requires that all nurses continue to develop their skills and knowledge through professional development and life-long learning (ANA, 2001). This requirement is also reflected in the nurse practice acts of many states and regulations across the globe. For example, Fowler (2011) noted in a British journal that nurses have a responsibility to themselves, their patients, and the profession to maintain and improve their knowledge because (a) nursing knowledge and practice is changing at a fast pace, (b) others look to nurses for up-to-date knowledge, (c) it is rewarding for nurses to know that they are using best practices, (d) nurses can't learn everything in school, and (e) promotions and career advancement require professional development. In addition, Cooper (2009) reported that meaningful professional development opportunities available to employees help the employer by increasing job satisfaction and making a more positive work environment. Both of these lead to improved retention of nurses. The overall message here is that professional development is *not* an option; it is a mandate for every nurse and should be supported by every employer.

Fowler (2012) stated that professional development is built on experience, education, and reflective practice. He noted that this takes time, but that time alone is not enough. Similar to Benner's (1984) novice-to-expert model, development doesn't occur by doing something over and over again, nor does it come by simply taking on new kinds of patients or procedures. Development requires that you seek additional education about how to improve what you are currently doing, as well as education about caring for different kinds of patients in different contexts. The ANA (2001) suggested that education could occur through networking with other professionals, peer review, attending continuing education sessions, reading professional publications, or going back to school. But there are other possibilities as well. Years ago, I worked with a group of fairly new nurses. We formed a journal club in order to increase our knowledge and to keep each other motivated to complete our readings. Most important, the journal club encouraged us to *think* about our nursing practice (this thinking is sometimes called *reflective practice*).

Reflective practice is poorly defined in the literature. Kinsella (2009) noted that a number of authors have complained that reflective practice was becoming a catch-all phrase, one that many thought they understood, but few could describe clearly. In her synthesis, Kinsella pointed out that reflective practice goes beyond knowing how to do something. Reflective practice focuses on the art of how something is done by bringing in the nurse's perspectives, observations, intuitions, and subtle adjustments to an activity to make it right for the individual patient. Reflective practice requires you to think about *how* you are doing what you are doing, and how it might or should be done *better* the next time. This is why our journal club was so helpful with our professional development activities. We read articles that presented evidence for a certain treatment or approach. At our meetings, we discussed and critiqued the information in the articles. We used our collective experiences and knowledge to explore how the information would apply in our setting and how we might alter it for different kinds of patients. Most important, we returned to the topic a month later. We shared whether or not the information changed our nursing practice. If it didn't, then why not? If it did, then how well did it work? What should be revised? If system problems prevented the change, how could we work for change in the system? Mantzoukas and Watkinson (2008) reported that some have stated that reflective practice contradicts evidence-based practice, especially the use of scientific methods and objectivity. In reality, both reflective practice and evidence-based practice are necessary. They are complimentary in nursing practice. In simpler terms, the art and science of nursing are not separate, but rather mixed together to make a more complete display of nursing practice. Experience shapes our perspectives and our nursing background. Education provides us the knowledge. Reflection marries the two in order to increase our understanding.

Professional development takes time. It does not happen immediately after reading a nursing article. Lack of time is one of the most common reasons nurses give for not engaging in professional development. To help, Fowler (2012) suggested that nurses consider professional development as a hobby, not as a chore. It's easier to schedule time for hobbies than for extra work. He also reminded us that professional development opportunities abound in the workplace. This makes professional development convenient. Expose yourself to unusual patients or procedures. Ask to be assigned to these patients, or have a discussion with staff who are assigned to these patients about their experiences. Attend all in-services and education offerings available to you at work. Discuss with your mentor the information from these offerings and how it might apply to your clinical practice.

Other barriers may make professional development more difficult. Schweitzer and Krassa (2010) reviewed ten studies and noted that in addition to time, nurses reported problems with cost of attending education offerings, distance to travel to offerings, and the inability to get time off of work. Some of these barriers can be minimized by seeking educational offerings online. Again, take the information you learn from these offerings and reflect on how it might apply to your own practice. Discuss your reflections with colleagues and mentors. Seek the guidance of clinical experts on the topic. Apply the information, as appropriate, and evaluate how well it worked.

Lou, Yu, and Chen (2010) completed an interesting study on male nurses in Taiwan. These researchers noted that male nurses in Taiwan were more interested in career advancement than were female nurses; therefore, more men were active in professional development. But not all men were actively involved. They surveyed 308 nurses and found that men who felt empowered were more likely to pursue professional development. A number of factors influence your sense of empowerment. Some factors come from the workplace (e.g., positive work setting, ability to make independent decisions about nursing care, respect from peers, and a culture that supports professional development). Other factors come from within (e.g., high level of personal accountability, good teamwork and collaboration skills, empathy, level of skill and knowledge, and positive self-esteem). Workplace factors may differ from setting to setting. If your workplace is not supportive of professional development, collaborate with your peers to make changes. Changing the workplace isn't always easy, but you must make some effort at this. After all, professional development is not an option for either you or the employer. On the other hand, you do have control over the internal forces. Professional development requires that you have the attributes of a professional. You were introduced to these while you were in nursing school. Remember them. Also, remember that one responsibility of a professional is to spend some of his own time and money in professional development activities. Just like it is your responsibility to make sure that your nursing license is current, it is your responsibility to make sure your knowledge and skill are current. Do not become one of the nurses I have met who have told me, "I'm not going to read journals if I don't get paid for it. When I'm off-the-clock, my time is mine. I don't do anything nursing on my own time." These nurses are not upholding the ethical code of the profession. These nurses are not true professionals.

FINDING A MENTOR

The best way to develop your professional knowledge and skill is to work with a mentor or group of mentors. Mentors have been used since ancient times. They help novices learn skills, but also how to navigate the culture of the workplace, develop problem-solving skills, and move forward with career advancement. Mentors are common in the world of business, but the use of formal mentors is relatively new in nursing. Still, few nurses seek mentors when they get their first job. Sure, new nurses ask for help and learn much from their coworkers, but a mentor is different from someone who simply helps you out. Having a mentor requires much thought and relationship building, but the benefits of having a mentor make your time and effort worthwhile. Carey and Weissman (2010) reported that protégés (people who have mentors) have increased confidence, job satisfaction, and professional development progress. You would be wise to seek a mentor once you have settled into your new job.

The word *mentor* sometimes is used interchangeably with the word *preceptor*. Although there is some overlap, these words refer to very different roles. Usually preceptors are assigned to you, whereas mentors are persons you chose. Preceptors are usually used when a person is new to a job. Mentors can be used any time after initial orientation, even if you have worked with the same employer for many years. The length of the relationship differs between a preceptor and a mentor. Usually you work with a preceptor for a short time. It may be a few weeks, though with residency programs, preceptors may work with you up to a year. These longer preceptor relationships may transition into mentor relationships. Mentors may stay with you for years. But the main difference between a preceptor and a mentor is the purpose of the relationship. Generally, preceptors help you transition into a new job and evaluate how well you transition to your new responsibilities. Mentors work more as professional coaches and advisors. Instead of telling you what to do, mentors guide your thinking so that you can see the right way more clearly. Mentors give you opportunities and challenges (Carey & Weissman, 2010). Like preceptors, mentors will teach and evaluate your performance, but the mentor's evaluation is more advisory in nature. Evaluations from mentors consist of feedback, advice, and constructive criticism. Their comments often are confidential. On the other hand, preceptors share their evaluation of your performance with your boss, who then decides if you are the right fit for the job.

Since mentor relationships may be long-term, you should choose your mentor or mentors wisely. The first step in choosing a mentor starts with you. First you must ask yourself, "What are my goals for having a mentor? What are my short-term and long-term career goals? What strengths do I already have? What needs and challenges do I see? What needs and challenges have others noticed in me?" Be clear about weak areas that may pose obstacles in reaching your goals. In thinking about possible mentors, you want to choose someone who will challenge you to work on your weaknesses. You want someone who will push you to go farther, deeper, and longer in your development. You do *not* want someone who will simply pat you on the back with congratulations. You want a mentor who will give a balanced mix of challenge and support. This mix will stimulate you to reflect, learn, and grow (Carey & Weissman, 2010).

When you have completed this self-examination, think about possible mentors. Ideally, mentors are recognized by others as leaders, good role models, team players, client advocates, and clinical experts. Good mentors are patient, dedicated to excellence, and successful in their own professional development. Good mentors have empathy and emotional intelligence. Keep in mind though, that real-life mentors are human, not fictitious heroes. No mentor will have every perfect mentor trait, so think about mentors who have the most important traits that will address your development needs. Then, look around. Let coworkers and professional contacts know that you are looking for a mentor. Make a possible list of mentors and contact them. Don't wait around for them to contact you. You must initiate the process. Make yourself attractive to a potential mentor by demonstrating your own dedication to excellence, openness to feedback, and professionalism. When approaching a possible mentor, be direct. Tell the potential mentor that you admire and respect his or her work. Share your needs and goals with the possible mentor and make your request, but then be sure to allow the potential mentor a way to gracefully decline your request. He or she may be too busy to serve as a mentor or may feel that he or she is not the right fit for your needs and goals. If this is the case, ask who might be recommended to serve as your mentor (Carey & Weissman, 2010; Laino-Curran, 1995; Sherwin, 2003).

Once someone agrees to serve as your mentor, Carey and Weissman (2010) suggested that it is *your* responsibility for maintaining the health of the relationship, not the mentor's. Start by learning the mentor's abilities and limitations, as well as the mentor's own needs. Mentors get pleasure out of helping out junior nurses, but mentors benefit in other ways. Mentors develop their own leadership and teaching skills when they mentor. Some mentors are able to make progress on their own projects when you provide your assistance. Becoming aware of the mentor's needs and goals will go far in making the relationship beneficial for both of you. Next, maintain a healthy relationship by always being prepared for your sessions with your mentor. If your mentor wants you to work on a case study or research the latest evidence on a treatment, complete this work well ahead of time. This will allow you the time to digest the information, reflect on your thoughts, and formulate questions. Preparation will show your mentor that you are committed to your professional development. Be on time when meeting with your mentor. This will show your mentor respect. Be open to feedback from your mentor, even if it is criticism. You cannot learn if you only hear what you are doing right. Maintain open and professional communication. Respect your mentor's privacy by keeping personal information confidential. Your mentor will do the same. And lastly, remember that your relationship with your mentor is a professional one. Becoming social friends with your mentor will blur the lines of the mentor role and may make it uncomfortable for him or her to give you honest feedback and guidance.

Relationships with mentors go through stages as do all relationships. There is the start of the relationship, in which you and your mentor get to know each other and agree on goals, meeting times, and scope of the relationship. Then, there is the maintenance of the relationship. During this stage, the professional development work you do may change as you advance or as goals and needs change. Then there is the ending of the relationship. Mentor relationships end for a number of reasons. Either you or the mentor may change jobs or move away so that the relationship cannot continue (although mentors can be effective even if they live thousands of miles away by using electronic ways to communicate with you). Either of you may have a sharp increase in workload or responsibilities, making it impossible to continue the relationship. There could be personality conflicts that could end the relationship. Or, a mentor relationship ends because the goals and needs have been met. In any case, either you or the mentor may choose to end the relationship. This choice should be respected gracefully (Carey & Weissman, 2010).

Finally, it is rare to find one mentor who will meet all your needs all at once, or meet all your needs over the life of your career. Often, nurses create a collection of different types of mentors. For example, you might choose a formal mentor that works as I have just described, but you might select a number of peer mentors as well. Peer mentors are colleagues who have about the same level of knowledge and professional development as you. Peer mentors can be effective confidantes and coaches. Sometimes people feel safer discussing their concerns with a peer than with someone who has more experience and power in an organization. Using peer mentors will help you develop networking and team building skills. At other times, you may choose a mosaic mentor model. This model includes two or more formal mentors, each helping you in different areas. For example, you may have a clinical mentor, a leadership mentor, and a research mentor all at the same time. And commonly, nurses have multiple mentors that come and go in a series. You may have a mentor as you develop your basic nursing clinical skills. Later, if you become a charge nurse, you may end the first mentor relationship and start a new relationship with a mentor who can help you develop administrative skills. Remember, the mentor pattern choice is yours, but chose a mentor for important times during your professional development journey. And as you advance to the next level of your career, pay your mentor back by mentoring those nurses that follow you.

LEADERSHIP

In my experience, nursing students often have confusing ideas about leadership. It's easy to understand why; many of us think about supervisors and administrators when we think about leaders in the work setting. Obviously these persons are leaders in rank and responsibility, but leadership is not unique to them. *Every* professional must understand leadership principles and display leadership behaviors. Health care consumers demand this. To start, I instruct students to become leaders of their own education. Students must evaluate their needs and explore necessary resources to improve their learning. As life-long learners, students graduate and must become leaders in their professional development as I have just discussed. As a registered nurse, you must develop leadership at the bedside, sometimes called *point-of-care* leadership. This type of leadership role requires you to take responsibility to ensure that the patient receives quality, safe, evidence-based care not only from you, but from other health team members as well. The nurse also becomes a gatekeeper and patient advocate. This leadership role falls upon your shoulders since the nurse is the one closest to the patient. The nurse knows the patient and spends more time with the patient than anyone else. Experts recognize this important relationship among nurses and their patients. Successful actions to improve the health care system can only occur if nurses at every level demonstrate leadership in the planning and delivery of health services (Adeniran, Bhattacharya, & Adeniran, 2012).

Today, we recognize that we must understand and display leadership differently than we had in the past. Until recently, rank and file employees were not required to display much leadership. Instead, they were expected to follow instructions and complete their work. Work emphasized completing a series of tasks that would ultimately accomplish a goal or create a product. The role of a leader was to make sure that the *process* worked efficiently. You can envision this as an assembly line in a factory. Porter-O'Grady and Malloch (2003) called this a Newtonian approach (after Isaac Newton, who viewed the universe as a large machine). If employers could make sure that the work process was efficient, the workplace (machine) would be productive and meet goals. This view created a system in which decisions come down from the top, work is tightly controlled with policies and rules, and employees were arranged in levels and hierarchies.

Early in the 20th century, scientists began to question the assumptions of Newton's machine-like view of the universe. For example, biologists could easily show how life doesn't work as predictably as a machine. A new view of science began to take shape called *quantum theory*, which recognizes irregularities and complex systems of actions. Porter-O'Grady and Malloch (2003) used this new theory as an analogy for the changes we need to make in how we view leadership. They called this new leadership *quantum leadership*. They noted that organizations, such as a health care setting, cannot be viewed like an assembly line. Instead, these organizations are a collection of multiple systems, such as various departments, groups of employees, groups of customers, and multiple services. These systems affect each other, often unpredictably. This makes sense if we look at a simple analogy. Think of your commute to work or school. You take a usual route and arrive at a consistent time. Today, the transportation department decides to start construction on the highway you take. On top of that, a driver gets distracted by texting her son and causes a chain reaction crash. Your predictable commute is now a mess, from systems that are external to you with which you have very little control. Quantum leadership requires that you understand systems and how systems work. Multiple systems, as we find in any work setting, are naturally complex. This complexity helps explain why unexpected things happen in organizations, or why changes don't always work simply because someone enforces new rules. Complexity seems to run amok, as if chaos ruled supreme. But loosely defined, chaos theory suggests that multiple systems have patterns that can be understood and managed. Patterns may have predictable consequences and adjustments, so that in reality, there is some order in the midst of chaos (Crowell, 2011). Going back to my traffic example, it could be predicted that construction would lead to traffic back-ups, which would increase the risk for accidents by distracted drivers. It could also be predicted that drivers would exit the highway and take side streets, causing further traffic snarls on other streets. The problems in this scene could be reduced with effective leadership and planning by the transportation department. Perhaps detours could have been created to relieve traffic, or construction planned to occur at night when traffic is lighter.

You must understand complexity in your work setting if you are to be a leader in your own nursing practice. Without this understanding, you will approach your work as if you simply need to check the tasks off of your daily list (Berwick, 2011). You must learn to see the big picture, that your actions sometimes do not lead to desired goals due to the influence of other systems. Gaining this understanding requires work, but is necessary if you are to learn how to alter your actions so that you can be effective working in complex systems. Adeniran et al. (2012) noted that mentorship and active professional development help new nurses understand the systems at play in their work setting. They further reported that nurses with self-efficacy, a belief that one has the ability to organize and execute actions that will reach goals, are better suited for systems understanding and leadership. Mentors can help you develop self-efficacy beliefs and skills.

However, simple awareness of complexity and systems is not enough to allow you to become a point-of-care leader. You need to understand the systems at play. Berwick (2011) instructed that nurses need to have in-depth knowledge about the variation and diversity encountered in health care. For example, healthy lab values don't always fall into normal ranges. Treatments don't always work the same for every individual. Patients often have different goals and priorities than their health care providers. Understanding and interpreting their variations are essential for quality care. Nurses also need better knowledge about psychology. Since systems in health care rarely operate independent of humans, nurses need to understand people, how people think and act, and how to work effectively with diverse groups of people. Also, nurses need better knowledge about knowledge, specifically, how to get information and how to use that information for complicated clinical decision-making.

Porter-O'Grady and Malloch (2003) proposed a set of skills that nurse leaders must develop. First, nurses must develop expertise at managing conflict. Conflict is natural and should be expected in any work setting. In order to manage conflict, nurses must understand human behavior, relationship building, and holding others accountable for working toward common goals. Next, each nurse must recognize and embrace his or her own vulnerabilities. There is value with this in that it allows you to take risks, stretch your capabilities, learn new knowledge, and cherish how you have grown. Vulnerability reduces the power of too much ego. Vulnerability fosters respect for diversity and open communication. Each nurse must learn to consider mistakes as opportunities for learning and improvement. For this to happen, nurses must also learn to recognize errors, analyze how errors occur, and how to respond to errors positively and appropriately. Next, nurses must develop emotional competence. This type of competence exhibits a high regard for others, a sense of justice and fairness, a willingness to take accountability, a willingness to address mistakes, and a willingness to take action when necessary. In order to develop this competence, nurses must understand the interconnections they have with others and value the unique creativity and contributions of others. It requires being open to new ideas, having compassion, and being optimistic. It also requires a tolerance for the ambiguities of the systems at play. Next, nurses must develop habits that will reduce bad behaviors that could poison healthy work relationships. Nurses must role model to self and others respectful and supportive teamwork, yet at the same time, hold others accountable for their bad behaviors. Holding others accountable does not include harsh criticism, but rather, supportive communication and problem-solving. Positive behaviors may go far in fostering a culture of hope, trust, energy, and goodwill. And lastly, nurses must be good to themselves. Leadership requires work. To be effective point-of-care leaders, nurses must tend to their own needs for rest, encouragement, and fulfillment.

SUMMARY

"Nurses eat their young" is a horrible saying that has been intimidating new nurses for years. It bothers me each time I hear it because it doesn't reflect today's reality. Sure, there are a few nurses out there who have little patience for novice nurses, or closer to the truth, feel very threatened by young, smart, and energetic nurses right out of school. Today, the challenges of transitioning from student to nurse rarely come from unwelcoming nurses. Instead, these challenges mostly come from system inadequacies and from the new nurse's lack of planning. The silver lining here is that there is much you can do to make your own transition smooth and successful.

Benner's model reminds us that we all enter practice just beyond the novice level for some skills, and deeply in the novice level in other skills when we graduate from school (Benner, 1984). Remember this. Do not assume that you enter practice well-prepared for a complex health care system no matter how well you did in school. Residency programs acknowledge this fact. These programs help guide the new nurse to learn and apply knowledge in a specific care setting. Confidence, clinical judgment, and problem-solving skills grow in these programs. Residency programs are fast becoming the norm, but if your employer does not offer a residency program, you can easily access information about the components of these programs and develop your own program in collaboration with your employer.

Success in a residency program and beyond depends a lot on you. You must understand and embrace the desire for professional development. Without this, you may never go beyond mid-level ability in Benner's model. Active participation in your own development benefits not only you, but your employer and your patients as well. Development takes time. It requires a combination of repeated and new clinical experiences, continuing education, and reflective practice. Many barriers can slow your development progress, but a development plan and the use of mentors can ensure that your progress continues to move forward.

Finally, if you are to truly excel in today's nursing, you must sharpen your leadership perspectives and skills. Nurses are no longer health care machines, busy completing tasks and following a multitude of orders. Today, nurses have greater responsibilities in assessing a health situation and creating an evidence-based plan of care that is developed in equal partnership with other health providers. Due to their close exposure to patients, nurses must be willing to fight for their patients' needs. Nurses must be the drivers of any change process if health care at the bedside is to improve in quality. In order to make this happen, you must become the leader of your own nursing practice. You must understand the complexity of the many systems working in your health setting. You must improve your ability to see the big picture, to understand how one action can have many consequences. Never before has nursing required so much of your sharp mind, your compassionate heart, and your healing hands. Never before has it been necessary for you to take such responsibility in developing your own nursing expertise. Never before has nursing been so exciting, challenging, and rewarding. Never before has it been a better time for you to be a nurse!

REFERENCES

Adeniran, R. K., Bhattacharya, A., & Adeniran, A. A. (2012). Professional excellence and career advancement in nursing: A conceptual framework for clinical leadership development. *Nursing Administration Quarterly, 36*(1), 41–51.

Altier, M. E., & Krsek, C. A. (2006). Effects of a 1-year residency program on job satisfaction and retention of new graduate nurses. *Journal for Nurses in Staff Development, 22*(2), 70–77.

American Nurses Association. (2001). *Code of ethics for nurses with interpretive statements*. Silver Spring, MD: Author.

Benner, P. (1984). *From novice to expert: Excellence and power in clinical nursing practice*. Menlo-Park, CA: Addison-Wesley.

Benner, P., Tanner, C., & Chesla, C.(Eds.). (2009). *Expertise in nursing practice: Caring, Clinical judgment, and ethics*. New York: Springer.

Benner, P., Sutphen, M., Leonard, V., & Day, L. (2010). *Educating nurses: A call for radical transformation:* San Francisco, CA: Jossey-Bass.

Berwick, D. M. (2011). Preparing nurses for participation in and leadership in continual improvement. *Journal of Nursing Education, 50*(6), 322–327.

Carey, E. C., & Weissman, D. E. (2010). Understanding and finding mentorship: A review for junior faculty. *Journal of Palliative Medicine, 13*(11), 1373–1379.

Cooper, E. (2009). Creating a culture of professional development: A milestone pathway tool for registered nurses. *The Journal of Continuing Education in Nursing, 40*(11), 501–507.

Crowell, D. M. (2011). *Complexity leadership: Nursing's role in health care delivery.* Philadelphia, PA: F. A. Davis.

Del Bueno, D. J. (2005). Why can't new registered nurse graduates think like nurses? *Nursing Education Perspectives, 26*(5), 278–282.

Duffield, C., Roche, M., O'Brien-Pallas, L., & Catling-Paull, C. (2009). The implication of staff 'churn' for nurse managers, staff, and patients. *Nurse Economics, 27*(2), 103–110.

Fowler, J. (2011). Professional development Part 1: The importance of professional development. *British Journal of Nursing, 20*(21), 1383.

Fowler, J. (2012). Professional development: From staff nurse to nurse consultant. Part 3: Making time. *British Journal of Nursing, 21*(1), 59.

Jones, C. B. (2008). Revisiting nurse turnover costs: Adjusting for inflation. *Journal of Nursing Administration, 38*(1), 11–18.

Kinsella, E. A. (2009). Professional knowledge and the epistemology of reflective practice. *Nursing Philosophy, 11*(1), 3–14.

Laino-Curran, D. (1995). Choosing your mentor: Finding your guide to a successful career. *Nursing, 25*(7), 78–79.

Lou, J., Yu, H., & Chen, S. (2010). Factors affecting the career development of male nurses: A structural equation model. *Journal of Advanced Nursing, 66*(4), 900–910.

Mantzoukas, S., & Watkinson, S. (2008). Redescribing reflective practice and evidence-based practice discourses. *International Journal of Nursing Practice, 14*(2), 129–134.

National Council of State Boards of Nursing. (2011). *Transition to practice.* Retrieved from http://www.ncsbn.org/363.htm

Porter-O'Grady, T., & Malloch, K. (2003). *Quantum leadership: A textbook of new leadership.* Sudbury, MA: Jones & Bartlett.

Schweitzer, D. J., & Krassa, T. J. (2010). Deterrents to nurses' participation in continuing professional development: An integrative literature review. *The Journal of Continuing Education in Nursing, 41*(10), 441–447.

Sherwin, L. N. (2003). Finding a mentor: What every nursing student should know. *Nursing News, 27*(3), 16.

Ulrich, B., Krozek, C., Early, S., Ashlock, C. H., Africa, L. M., & Carman, M. L. (2010). Improving retention and competence of new graduate nurses: Results from a 10-year longitudinal database. *Nursing Economics, 28*(6), 363–375.

Index